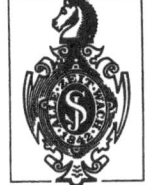

Controversies in
Cardiac
Rehabilitation

Edited by P. Mathes and M.J. Halhuber

With 87 Figures and 48 Tables

Springer-Verlag
Berlin Heidelberg New York 1982

Professor Dr. Peter Mathes
Professor Dr. Max J. Halhuber

Klinik Höhenried für Herz- und Kreislauferkrankungen
D-8131 Bernried/Obb., Germany

ISBN-13: 978-3-642-68381-7   e-ISBN-13: 978-3-642-68379-4
DOI: 10.1007/978-3-642-68379-4

Library of Congress Cataloging in Publication Data. Main entry under Title: Controversies
in cardiac rehabilitation. Bibliography: p. Includes index. 1. Cardiacs–Rehabilitation–
Congresses. I. Mathes, P. (Peter), 1940-. II. Halhuber, M.J. (Max Josef), 1916-. [DNLM: 1.
Coronary disease–Rehabilitation–Congresses. 2. Myocardial infarction–Rehabilitation–
Congresses. WG 300 C764 1982] RC682.C66 616.1'206 81-21287 AACR2

2121/3140-543210

Preface

This book contains the proceedings of a conference organized by the Klinik Höhenried at the Evangelische Akademie in Tutzing under the patronage of the International Society of Cardiology — Council on Rehabilitation — from Febr. 12–14, 1981.

The purpose of the meeting on Current Problems in Cardiac Rehabilitation was to come closer to answering the questions posed in the following pages, and to make some opinions about cardiac rehabilitation less contoversial. To comment briefly on the interesting question of why opinions in the field of cardiac rehabilitation seem more controversial than in other fields of cardiology, we would like to propose the following explanation:

1. Lack of personal experience and lack of special training in cardiac rehabilitation are a major source of misunderstandings and differences of vocabulary between cardiologists engaged in clinical practice and in rehabilitation.
2. Emotional problems in accepting a new kind of partnership between coronary patients and their physicians and a "nihilistic attitude" towards therapy of behaviour play an important role in the scepticism of cardiologists.
3. Fear of an expensive "overmedication" (I. Illich) is another argument concerning rehabilitation.
4. Lack of controlled studies in this new field may give a valid reason for criticism. However, the problems of methodology are not yet resolved. In many Western countries controlled long-term studies of chronic diseases which depend on behaviour patterns frequently suffer from methodological difficulties. Just one example is that there may be as many "drop-ins" from the control group into the experimental group with intervention measures as there are "drop-outs". For studies in cardiac rehabilitation today we need an interdisciplinary ecological approach and as a background to such an approach we need new scientific theories of methodology.
5. Finally, semantic problems in defining terms, and therefore many misunderstandings of "rehabilitation", are more common than we believe. A generally accepted theory of cardiac rehabilitation as an interdisciplinary science exists only in outline. Everbody has his own philosophy, which is often an ideology (i.e. an interpretation of the world which is deeply influenced by interests).

We would like to express our appreciation for the generous support of the meeting and the proceedings by Pharma-Schwarz Company,

Monheim, West-Germany. We also would like to thank all authors of this book for their contibution and to the Springer-Verlag, Heidelberg, for a careful edition.

Prof. M.J. Halhuber
Prof. P. Mathes

Contents

List of Contributors

-

Prof. Dr. W.E. Adam
Universität Ulm, Abteilung Radiologie III, Steinhövelstraße 9, D-7900
Ulm, Germany

Prof. Dr. K. Bachmann
Universität Erlangen-Nürnberg, Medizinische Poliklinik, Östliche Stadt-
mauer-Strasse 29, D-8520 Erlangen, Germany

Dr. K.-P. Bethge
Medizinische Hochschule Hannover, Department Innere Medizin, Ab-
teilung Kardiologie, Karl-Wiechert-Allee 9, D-3000 Hannover 61,
Germany

Dr. F. Bitter
Universität Ulm, Abteilung Radiologie III, Steinhövelstrasse 9, D-7900
Ulm, Germany

P. Block, M.D.
Thoraxcenter Erasmus University, Post Box 1738, NL-3000 DR Rotterdam, The Netherlands

Prof. Dr. G. Blümchen
Klinik Roderbirken, Fachklinik für Herz- und Kreislauferkrankungen,
D-5653 Leichingen 1, Germany

M.G. Bourassa, M.D.
47 Marechal Exelmans, F-54000 Nancy, France

B. Caru, M.D.
Centro de Gasperis, Ospedale Maggiore, I-20251 Milano, Italy

Dr. G. Czerwenka-Wenkstetten
Medizinische Universitätsklinik, Allgemeines Krankenhaus der Stadt
Wien, Garnisonsgasse 13, A-1097 Wien, Austria

N. Danchin, M.D.
Centre Hospitalier Regional de Nancy, Hopital de Brabois, 5400
Vandoerre-Lès-Nancy

P. David, M.D.
Institut de Cardiologie de Montreal, 5000 Est, Rue Belanger, Montreal,
Quebec, Canada

Dr. A. Eder
Medizinische Universitätsklinik, Allgemeines Krankenhaus der Stadt
Wien, Garnisonsgasse 13, A-1097 Wien, Austria

Prof. Dr. J. von der Emde
Universitätsklinik, Herzchirurgische Abteilung, Maximiliansplatz, D-
8520 Erlangen, Germany

Prof. Dr. F.H. Epstein
Universität Zürich, Institut für Sozial- und Präventivmedizin, Gloria-
strasse 32, CH-8006 Zürich, Switzerland

Dr. L. Görnandt
Benedikt Kreutz-Rehabilitationszentrum für Herz- und Kreislauf-
kranke, Südring 15, D-7812 Bad Krozingen, Germany

Dr. H. Gohlke
Benedikt Kreutz-Rehabilitationszentrum für Herz- und Kreislauf-
kranke, Südring 15, D-7812 Bad Krozingen, Germany

Prof. P. Hackett, M.D.
Massachusetts General Hospital, Boston, MA 02114, USA

Prof. Dr. M.J. Halhuber
Klinik Höhenried für Herz- und Kreislaufkrankheiten, D-8139 Bernried/
Obb., Germany

Prof. Dr. G. Hartmann
Medizinische Klinik, Kantonsspital, CH-7000 Chur, Switzerland

Dr. K. Heidecker
Benedikt Kreutz-Rehabilitationszentrum für Herz- und Kreislauf-
kranke, Südring 15, D-7812 Bad Krozingen, Germany

Prof. Dr. W. Hollmann
Deutsche Sporthochschule Köln, Institut für Kreislaufforschung und
Sportmedizin, Carl-Diem-Weg, D-5000 Köln 41, Germany

Prof. P.G. Hugenholtz, M.D.
Thoraxcenter/Cardiology, Academisch Ziekenhuis, Dr. Molewater-
plein 40, NL-3015 GD Rotterdam, The Netherlands

Prof. T. Kavanagh, M.D.
Toronto Rehabilitation Centre, 345 Rumsey Road, Toronto, Ontario,
M4 & 1R7, Canada

Prof. J.J. Kellermann, M.D.
Cardiac Evaluation and Rehabilitation Institut, The Chaim Sheba
Medical Center, Tel-Hashomer, Israel

Prof. Dr. K. König
Fachklinik für Herzkreislauferkrankungen, Kandelstrasse 41, D-7808
Waldkirch/Freiburg, Germany

M. Kornitzer, M.D.
Ecole de Sante Publique, Campus Erasme-CP 590, Route de Lennik
808, B-1070 Bruxelles, Belgium

Dr. B. Krug
Medizinische Universitätsklinik, Sigmund Freud-Strasse 25, B-5300
Bonn-Venusberg, Germany

Prof. Dr. P.R. Lichtlen
Medizinische Hochschule Hannover, Department Innere Medizin,
Abteilung Kardiologie, Karl-Wiechert-Allee 9, D-3000 Hannover 61,
Germany

Prof. B. Lown, M.D.
Harvard University, School of Public Health, 665 Huntington Avenue,
Boston, MA 02115, USA

Prof. P. Mathes
Klinik Höhenried für Herz- und Kreislaufkrankheiten, D-8139 Bernried/
Obb., Germany

R.S. Meltzer, M.D.
Thoraxcenter Erasmus University, Post Box 1738, NL-3000 DR Rotterdam, The Netherlands

Prof. R. Mulcahy, M.D., F.R.C.P., F.R.C.P.I.
The Sisters of Charity, St. Vincent's Hospital, Elm Park, Dublin 4,
Ireland

Doz. Dr. M. Niederberger
Medizinische Universitätsklinik, Allgemeines Krankenhaus der Stadt
Wien, Garnisonsgasse 13, A-1097 Wien, Austria

P. Robert, M.D.
Institut de Cardiologie de Montreal, 5000 Est, Rue Belanger, Montreal,
Quebec, Canada

J. Roeland, M.D.
Thoraxcenter Erasmus University, Post Box 1738, NL-3000 DR Rotterdam, The Netherlands

Prof. Dr. H. Roskamm
Benedikt Kreutz-Rehabilitationszentrum für Herz- und Kreislauf-
kranke, Südring 15, D-7812 Bad Krozingen, Germany

Prof. Dr. R. Rost
Deutsche Sporthochschule Köln, Institut für Kreislaufforschung und
Sportmedizin, Carl-Diem-Weg, D-5000 Köln 41, Germany

Dr. H. Rüddel
Medizinische Universitätsklinik, Sigmund Freud-Straße 25, D-5300
Bonn-Venusberg, Germany

Dr. L. Samek
Benedikt Kreutz-Rehabilitationszentrum für Herz- und Kreislauf-
kranke, Südring 15, D-7812 Bad Krozingen, Germany

Dr. G. Schilling
Medizinische Universitätsklinik, Sigmund Freud-Strasse 25, D-5300
Bonn-Venusberg, Germany

Dr. K. Schnellbacher
Benedikt Kreutz-Rehabilitationszentrum für Herz- und Kreislauf-
kranke, Südring 15, D-7812 Bad Krozingen, Germany

Dr. A. Schöneberger
Klinikum der Universität, Zentrum der Inneren Medizin, Abteilung für
Kardiologie, Theodor-Stern-Kai 7, D-6000 Frankfurt/M. 70, Germany

Prof. Dr. J. Siegrist
Medizinische Soziologie, Robert-Koch-Strasse 7, D-3550 Marburg/
Lahn, Germany

Prof. Dr. H. Simon
Medizinische Universitätsklinik, Sigmund Freud-Strasse 25, D-5300
Bonn-Venusberg, Germany

M.L. Simoons, M.D.
Thoraxcenter Erasmus University, Post Box 1738, NL-3000 DR Rotterdam, The Netherlands

Prof. Dr. M. Stauch
Universität Ulm, Abteilung Radiologie III, Steinhövelstrasse 9, D-7900
Ulm, Germany

Dr. P. Stürzenhofecker
Benedikt Kreutz-Rehabilitationszentrum für Herz- und Kreislauf-
kranke, Südring 15, D-7812 Bad Krozingen, Germany

Dr. R.L. Verrier
Harvard University, Department of Public Health, 665 Huntington
Avenue, Boston, Mass. 02115, USA

Prof. N.K. Wenger, M.D.
Emory University School of Medicine, Grady Memorial Hospital, 69
Butler Street, S.E., Atlanta, GA 30303, USA

Prof. Dr. L. Wilhelmsen
Östra Hospital, Department of Medicine, Plan 2, S-416-85 Göteborg,
Sweden

The Role of Diet

G. Hartmann

The identification of risk factors and their modification are essential whenever we aim at primary or secondary prevention of coronary heart disease. We have a heavy commitment to do so considering the frequency and malignancy of the disease. If we think of those 30%—40% of patients who die within 2 days after myocardial infarction, it is evident that its seriousness has been considerably underestimated.

As there is still no means of curing coronary heart disease, we are confined to alleviating symptoms and complications. Mindful of this hard fact, preventive measures are of paramount importance. Opinions differ whether we have to strain for all available and acceptable measures or rely only on those which have proven absolutely effective over many years and for any given situation.

Although knowledge has increased remarkably over the last 20 years, the genesis of atherosclerosis and coronary heart disease ist still poorly understood, very complex, but certainly multifactorial. The latter aspect contributed most to the issue of prevention. It is the origin of the concept of multiple risk factors, widely accepted today.

Nutrition plays a key role in the management of the crucial, well-established coronary risk factors as shown in the following list:

> Hyperlipidemia
> Cigarette smoking
> Hypertension
> Diabetes mellitus
> Physical inactivity
> Psychosocial stress
> Overweight
> Heredity

Its priority in controlling overweight and diabetes is unequivocal, and it is also of primary importance in hypertension.

However, the main impact of diet is on the risk factor hyperlipidemia, which itself plays a key role in the whole issue. This relationship, involving both cholesterol and triglycerides or different lipoproteins, is the core of the "Diet/Heart-Question" and has often been the subject of controvery. Is there any reason for this?

The validity of the theory that hyperlipidemia plays the leading role in atherogenesis and coronary heart disease is so well established that it cannot be repudiated [1—4]. While the main body of data is well known (Table 1), a few important results of the prospective Basel

Table 1. Findings supporting the lipid theory of CHD

Experimental	Superiority of fat feeding for AS
Angiochemistry	Lipids corresponding to plasma pattern
Epidemiologic	Correlation to fat intake
	Correlation to serum cholesterol
Clinical	MI increase with plasma lipids
	Angiographic stenosis correlates to serum lipids
	OPAD more frequent with higher lipids
	Juvenile MI in homozygous type II-A
	MI increased in secondary hyperlipidemias
Therapeutic	Regression xanthomas by lipid lowering
	Regression CHD by lipid lowering (?)

AS, atherosclerosis
MI, myocardial infarction
OPAD, occlusive peripheral arterial disease

Study are presented, which have only been published in part [5]. It can easily be shown that the almost linear relationship between serum cholesterol and the incidence of myocardial infarction is also valid in Switzerland (Fig. 1). Cardiac death is also more frequent with higher cholesterol and triglycerides levels (Fig. 2). There are arguments which favour even an independent prospective significance of triglycerides [5].

The relationship between nutrition and serum lipids is manifold and documented by a vast amount of literature. We want to summarize briefly the influence of nutrition on cholesterol or LDL particles as well as on triglycerides or VLDL. At least six parameters of the diet are responsible for the cholesterol concentration of any normal person:

> Total calories
> Fat calories
> Saturated fat
> P/S ratio
> Cholesterol
> Fiber
> Protein

According to Lewis [6] the maximal effects achievable are around 50 mg/dl as shown in the following list:

Reduced and modified fat intake (30%, P/S 1.0)	− 20 mg/dl
Reduced cholesterol intake (200 mg)	− 8 mg/dl
Increased fibre intake (6 → 46 g)	− 16 mg/dl
Modified protein intake (vegetable ↑)	− 8 mg/dl
Sum △ cholesterol	− 51 mg/dl

Factors influencing triglycerides are less numerous and not easily quantifiable:

> Total calories

Carbohydrate calories
Carbohydrate type
Ethanol

The point is that we actually know quite well how to manipulate serum liquids by diet, but the practical application of this knowledge in terms of mass prevention brings a lot of problems. Indeed, controversies have arisen from attempts to lower lipids by dietary means on a large scale. Some doubt the benefit [7], while others question the practical value of recommendations [8]. However critical we may be, the very approach is largely a matter of personal opinion.

Those who are requesting statistical evidence may have to wait many years to get it. We cannot ignore the fact that the pathogenesis of the atherosclerotic lesions is very complex and that this process ovbiously takes decades. That makes it extraordinarily difficult to obtain

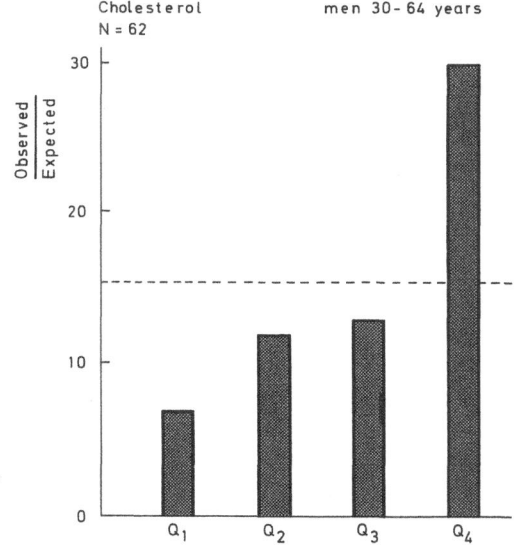

Fig. 1. Quartiles for cholesterol *(observed/expected cases)* in non-fatal myocardial infarction (Basel Study)

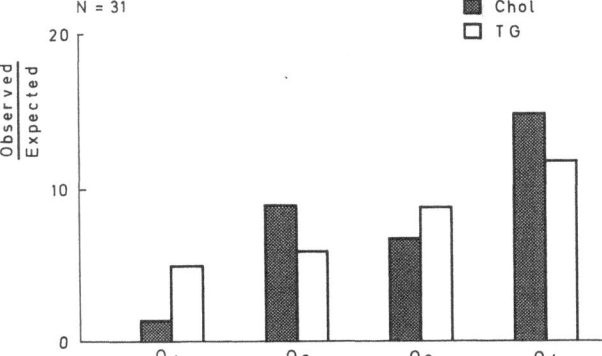

Fig. 2. Quartiles for cholesterol and triglycerides *(TG) (observed/expected cases)* in myocardial deaths (Basel Study)

conclusive evidence for interventions on single factors like cholesterol, which will reduce morbidity and mortality of myocardial infarction.

Certainly cholesterol or lipids are only one of several factors involved in myocardial infarction, but there are very impressive indications of the benefits resulting from their use as interventional measures in myocardial infarction, a few being as follows:

1. Lipid lowering by diet or drugs induces mobilization of tissue cholesterol (personal documentation).
2. The WHO clofibrate study has shown a 20% decrease in CHD morbidity by reducing cholesterol over 5 years by only 9% on average [9].
3. Recent publications give evidence that successful lipid lowering can prevent progression of angiographically documented atherosclerosis, or even induce regression [10, 11].

It is not only our personal opinion that diet in lowering lipids has the same rational basis as the control of hyperglycemia in diabetes [12], which is generally accepted. In addition, diet has practically no side effects. But it is essential to concentrate treatment and advice on the right target group. We experienced some controversy because theoretically correct recommendations were made indiscriminately, ignoring necessity and the ability of people to follow them. It happened because feasibility was neglected, impeding in this way the potential and desired success. Moreover it provoked opponents in the commercial field.

We have to bear in mind that the problem is more complex than preventing rickets. Having butter or margarine for breakfast is not the major issue when considering the long-term effect on serum cholesterol. If we want to bring about a change, we have to:

1. Cut saturated fats drastically.
2. Reduce calories.
3. Increase the P/S ratio.

How difficult this task will be can be seen from our experience with patients with type II hyperlipidemia. The most we can achieve is a reduction of 10%–15% for cholesterol [11]. With this in mind, we are reluctant to make generalized recommendations.

In conclusion dietary measures aimed at preventing CHD have to concentrate on selected patients and definite risk groups. By means of caloric restrictions, reduction of saturated fats and fat exchange, we can achieve success with cooperative people. But we have to check in any individual whether these measurements are really necessary and whether they do indeed have a chance of succeeding.

We shall have no controversies if we apply established scientific knowledge to the right people using common sense.

References

1   Levy RI (1980) Dietary prevention of coronary artery disease. A policy overview. In: Gotto AM Jr, Smith LC, Allen B (eds) Atherosclerosis V. Springer, Berlin Heidelberg New York, p 199
2   Stamler J (1980) The established relationship among diet, serum cholesterol and coronary heart disease. Acta Med Scand 207:433
3   Epstein FH, Gutzwiller F, Howald H, Junod B, Schweizer W (1979) Prävention der Atherosklerose: Grundlagen heute. Schweiz Med Wochenschr 109:1171

4 The Pooling Project Research Group (1978) Relationship of blood pressure, serum cholesterol, smoking habit, relative weight and ECG abnormalities to incidence of major coronary events. J Chronic Dis 31:201

5 Hartmann G, Stähelin HB (1980) Hyperlipidämie und Atherosklerose in der Schweiz: Ergebnisse aus der Basler Studie. Ther Umsch 37:980

6 Lewis B (1978) Hypothesis into theory − The development of aetiological concepts of ischaemic heart disease: A review. J R Soc Med 71:809−818

7 Werkö L (1979) Diet, lipids and heart attacks (Editorial). Acta Med Scand 206:435

8 Ahrens EH (1979) Dietary fats and coronary heart disease: Unfinished business. Lancet II:1345

9 Committee of Principal Investigators (1978) A co-operative trial in the primary prevention of ischaemic heart disease using clofibrate. Br Heart J 40:1069

10 Barndt R, Blankenhorn DH, Crawford DW, Brooks SH (1977) Regression and progression of early femoral atherosclerosis in treated hyperlipoproteinemic patients. Ann Intern Med 86:139

11 Thompson GH, Kilpatrick D, Oakley C, Stiener R, Myant N (1978) Reversal of cholesterolemia by long term plasma exchange. Circulation [Suppl 2] 58:171

12 Schlierf G, Oster P (1980) Diättherapie der Hyperlipoproteinämien. Ther Umsch 37:985

The Role of Social Factors — Behavior Patterns or Risk Situations?

J. Siegrist

This paper will focus on three questions: First (and in a very abbreviated manner): What are in general terms the probable links between psychosocial risks and coronary heart disease (CHD)?

Second: How can we define psychosocial stress in an operational way which fits into general scientific criteria?

Third: Is there as yet any evidence for such a concept from sociomedical research? And what are the main open questions?

Turning to the first question, I should like to distinguish analytically three possible pathways relating social, environmental, and personal traits to the development of CHD.

1. It is well established that some of the traditional risk factors, such as smoking, lack of physical exercise, and faulty diet, are related to specific sociocultural, socioeconomic, and/or psychological traits. Even if the relation between social factors and CHD is an indirect one, effective intervention and treatment of the disease has to take into account these influences and forces which may reinforce ill-health behavior.

2. One of the most important traditional risk factors, high blood pressure, has been linked experimentally and clinically to higher nervous activity: an increase in blood pressure can be regarded as a consequence of an arousal of the sympathetic-adrenomedullary system, specifically as a consequence of stimulation of angiotension II, ADH, and cate-cholamines (Ganten 1980). The role of these neurohormonal substances in the development of essential hypertension is still controversial (Birkenhäger and Falge 1978; Galosy and Gaebelein 1977), but experimental work (Folkow 1975; Henry and Stephens 1977) and epidemiologic studies on air-traffic controllers (Cobb and Rose 1973) and on workers with noise exposure (Kavoussi 1973; Suvorov et al. 1979) reinforce the hypothesis.

3. The traditional well-known factors explain — in terms of multivariate statistical analysis — about 60% of the observed variance in prospective studies (Epstein 1979). What about the many escapers and the paradoxical cases? It is possible that some somatic factor which has still to be detected may operate as a common denominator. It is also possible — and this is my hypothesis — that continuous or excessive stimulation of higher nervous activity by certain social and/or psychological factors may trigger pathological changes in the cardiovascular system. In this context we have to distinguish long-term and short-term effects. The best evidence, until now, has been established in the area of short-term effects, especially of ventricular premature beats and arrhythmias (Lown et al. 1977). Recent observations on the role of endorphines as secondary triggers in situations of neurohormonal imbalance which may disrupt vital functioning and cause heart failure and sudden death deserve special attention (Kordon 1980, personal communication). Coronary spasm is being increasingly reported in persons with premature myocardial infarction. Long-term influences have been discussed with regard, among other things, to deleterious effects of CNS-stimulated glucocorticoids on myocardial metabolism (Raab 1970; Selye 1976), to mobilization of blood lipids (Taggard et al. 1971), and to an increased demand of oxygen by sympathetic arousal.

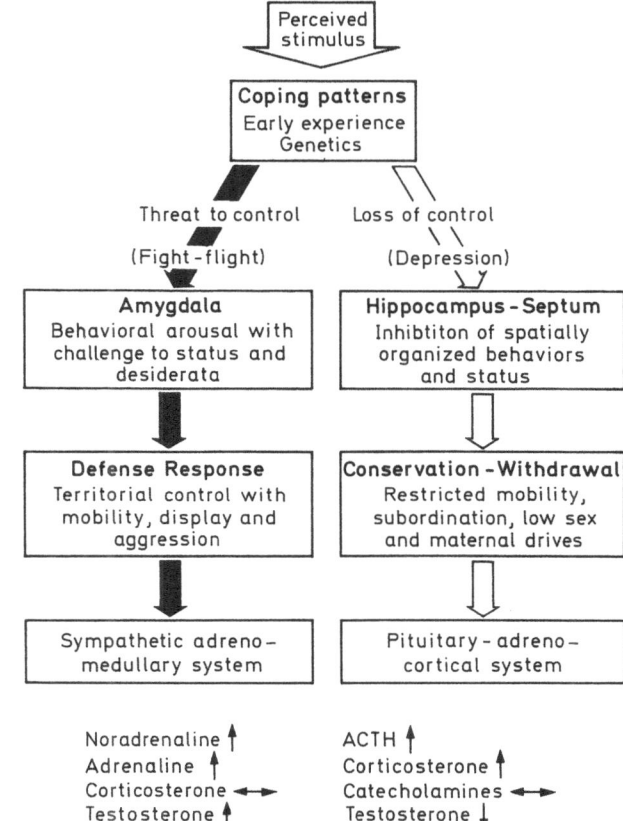

Fig. 1. Perceived stress and different neuroendocrine reaction patterns (Henry and Stephens 1977)

Summing up this information we can conclude that there is a reasonable basis for more fundamental research in an interdisciplinary field including psychosociology, neuroendocrinology, and pathophysiology of CHD.

How can we draw a concept and measure psychosocial influences involved in these processes? I shall give at least a preliminary answer to the second question. My answer has been heavily influenced by the work of Henry and Stephens (1977) and of Frankenhaeuser (1979, 1980). Both morphologically and functionally we can distinguish two neuroendocrine mechanisms which are involved in coping with stressful events: the sympathetic-adrenomedullary system, with the secretion of catecholamines (among other substances) and the pituitary-adrenocortical system, with the secretion of cortical steroids (among other substances). Animal research has suggested that these two reactions may be attributed to environmental influences in relation to the degree of control an individual possesses over this situation: active control over a stressor enhances the well-known fight-flight reaction first described by Cannon, whereas loss of control stimulates the conservation-withdrawal reaction detected by Selye. Experimental psychophysiologic work has shown that we have to take into account not only properties of the environmental stimulus but also the cognitive appraisal of "the balance between the severity of the situational demands and the personal coping resources" (Frankenhaeuser, to be published). It follows from this argument that we can distinguish three patterns of stress:

1. Demanding situations which are accompanied by effective coping and a feeling of mastery activate the sympathetic system with release of catecholamines, but only during exposure. This pattern may be labeled *eustress*.
2. Demanding situations which are accompanied by ineffective coping and by feelings of inadequacy, failure, self-punishment or hostility have been shown to activate both neuro-endocrine systems and to produce excessive catecholamine and cortisol release during a longer time period. This pattern may be labeled *active distress*.
3. Situations which induce a loss of control without any effort to act and which are associated with feelings of helpnessness produce a marked and prolonged elevation of cortico-steroid release. This pattern may be labeled *passive distress*.

From these considerations we can conclude that psychosocial risks of coronary heart disease are mainly due to the second pattern, namely active distress. Active distress is a specific pattern of neuroendocrine reaction to a specific person-environment interaction which can be defined as a discrepancy between situational demands and coping resources. Emotionally this discrepancy is answered by feelings of inadequacy, failure or hostility. This operational definition includes three types of information — endocrinological (hormones), psychological (persons), and sociological (social situations) — which have to be combined in meaningful measures.

The last question to be answered here relates to current research on this specific person-environment interaction which causes active distress. Until recently much research focused on a single personal trait, namely the coronary-prone behavior pattern (also called type A behavior) which, by and large, has been conceptualized as a stable personality trait (Dembroski and Halhuber, to be published). In a new publication the social psychologist David Glass argues against this position: "Serious considerations should be given to the notion that type A behavior is an outgrowth of a person-situation interaction. Efforts need to be directed towards the delineation of the classes of environmental stimuli that elicit the primary facets of the behavior pattern" (Glass 1981).

In a controlled retrospective study of 380 male patients (age 30–55) with a clinically documented first myocardial infarction who were participating in a rehabilitation program and a healthy control group matched with the sample half on the basis of age and occupation, we were able to find empirical evidence for this perspective. The 380 myocardial infarction patients were studied again 18 months later by means of a questionnaire focusing on occupational, medical, and psychosocial rehabilitation. The following hypotheses have been tested:

1. Type A is significantly higher in professional groups characterized by high work demand and limited autonomy than in professional groups characterized by monotonous industrial work.
2. The extent of type A within the same person changes over time as a result of challenges and difficulties in the occupational field.
3. Patients with premature myocardial infarction show significantly more psychosocial risk constellations in the premorbid period than healthy controls. Simultaneous presence of risk disposition (type A) and risk situations (work load, family conflicts, loss of social support) as well as combinations of chronic difficulties and subacute life-events are much more common among them.

4. These psychosocial risk constellations are also relevant as predictors for cardiac rehabilitation: psychosocial high risk conditions are much more probable in persons with cardiac death and/or recurrence of cardiac symptoms.

The first hypothesis was studied by contrasting two homogeneous occupational subgroups with respect to their mean type A values: on the one hand the subgroup of middle-echelon employees (supervisors and factory foremen) whose work places were characterized by inconsistent demands and limited room for decision, on the other hand the blue-collar industrial worker with rather simple, monotonous work demands. In both myocardial infarction patients and healthy controls, the middle-echelon employees had higher mean type A scores (statistically significant at the 0.01 level in the myocardial infarction population only) (Fig. 2).

Second hypothesis: In our study we found that the mean of type A scores increased significantly ($P < 0.01$) 18 months after the first screening. The percentage of persons with extremely high scores had nearly doubled. Interestingly, persons with the greatest amount of actual strain in the field of work and health showed the highest degree of type A behavior (N, 244: C, 0.45; $P < 0.001$) (Fig. 3).

Third hypothesis: If we look at the three most important psychosocial indices separately [work-load, life-events, and ambitions of control (type A)], we may recognize highly significant differences in mean values in each of them. However, if we combine the three variables in a common unweighted index, a much greater difference in the mean values can be recognized. The same result becomes even more obvious if we compare the extreme groups: the high risk group which in all three respects, i.e., work-load, life-events, and

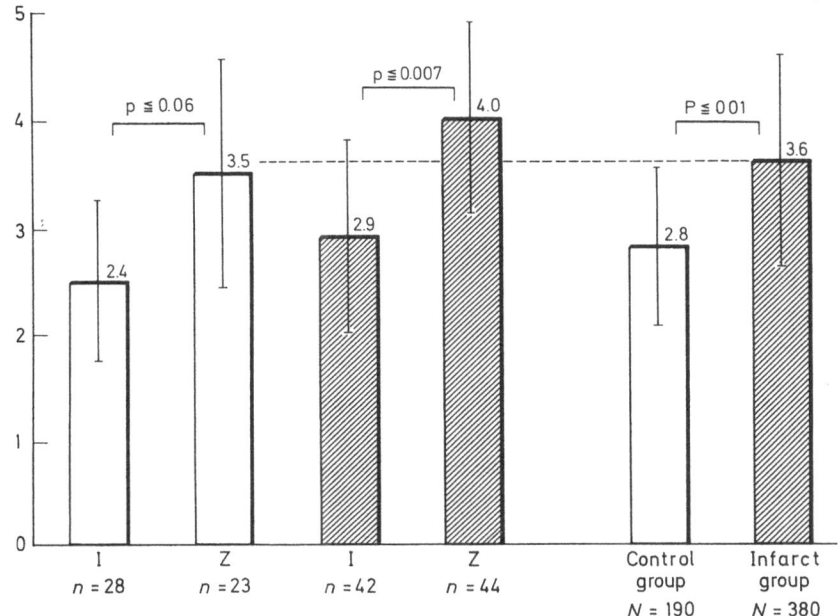

Fig. 2. Relations between ambitions of control (type A) and professional groups (Siegrist et al. 1980). I, blue-collar workers (industry; Z, middle-echelon employees; ☐ , healthy controls; ▨ , MI patients)

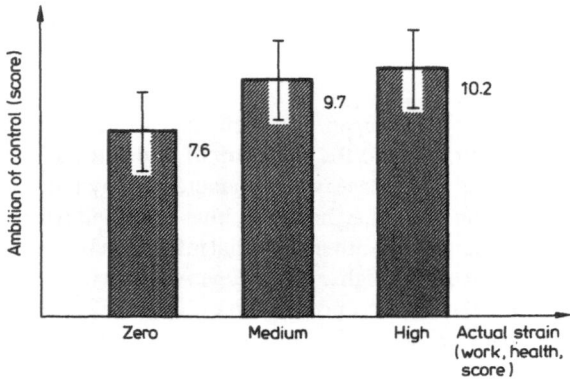

Fig. 3. Extent of ambitions of control (type A) in relation to actual strain in post-infarct patients (*N*, 244; *C*, 0.45; *p* < 0.001) (Siegrist et al. 1980)

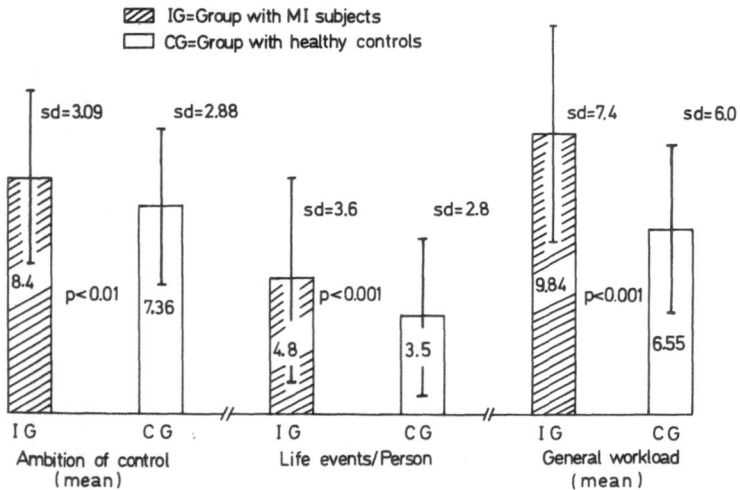

Fig. 4. Single stress indicators (N = 190) (Siegrist et al. 1980)

ambitions of control, is associated with extremely high values, can be found 4.3 times more often in myocardial infarction patients than in healthy individuals. In contrast the low risk group, whose values in all three categories are zero or close to zero, is twice as prevalent in healthy individuals compared to infarct patients. It is of special interest that denial, measured by a subscale of MMPI, is significantly higher among low risk myocardial infarction persons than among the high risk group (Fig. 4 and 5).

A step-wise discriminant analysis leads to similar results. Some 70%—75% of myocardial infarction patients and controls are correctly classified, mainly by psychosocial risk factors. In addition, we found a systematic relationship between the extent of chronic difficulties and subacute life-events in the field of family conflicts as well as in the field of work-load (Table 1 and 2).

High risk versus low risk group

N = 190   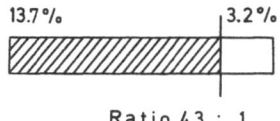 = IG

Low risk / CG

High workload + high life events + high ambitions of control:

13.7 %   3.2 %

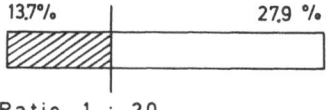

Ratio 4.3 : 1

Low workload + low life events + low ambitions of control:

13,7%   27,9 %

Ratio 1 : 2,0

Fig. 5. Extreme groups with psycho-social risks (Siegrist et al. 1980)

Fourth hypothesis: Evidence for an accumulation of chronic and subacute stress was demonstrated in our catamnestic study, including 324 of the initial 380 myocardial infarction patients. In the meantime 13 patients died of a second infarction. Figure 6 shows the presence of social risk situations in healthy individuals, in surviving myocardial infarction patients, and in those individuals who died in the meantime. High occupational stress and/or high life-event values are indicated in the upper diagram, and high occupational stress only, in the lower one. The percentage of those subjected to high degrees of stress among those who died in the meantime, in both cases, is more than twice the percentage observed in the healthy individuals. A smaller, but still obvious difference existed in comparison with surviving myocardial infarction patients. It is important to mention that only two of the 13 deceased patients were clinically characterized either by angiographically documented significant (> 50%) narrowing of two or three vessels or by ischemic ST depressions in exercise ECG below 50 W.

Let me conclude by saying that there is growing evidence linking psychosocial factors to CHD. But basic problems still need to be resolved. One of them has been identified by the cardiologist Kornitzer: "The crucial test of relating blood or urinary catecholamine levels

Table 1. Stepwise discriminant analysis (N = 190 MI subjects and 190 healthy controls), (Siegrist et al. 1980)

Actual group	Predicted group membership			
	MI subjects		Healthy controls	
MI subjects	134	70,5%	56	29,5%
Healthy controls	52	27,4%	138	72,6%

Percent of cases correctly classified: 71,6%

Table 2. Relations between chronic familial difficulties and live event scores (Analysis of variance); N = 380 MI subjects (Siegrist et al. 1980)

Chronic difficulty	Life event score		
	F : p		t-test : p
Marital conflicts	8.173	0.001	0.01
Problems with children	19.015	0.001	0.01
Trouble with neighbors	2.873	0.05	0.01
Difficulties with people in general	37.310	0.001	0.01
Bad housing situation	7.434	0.001	0.01

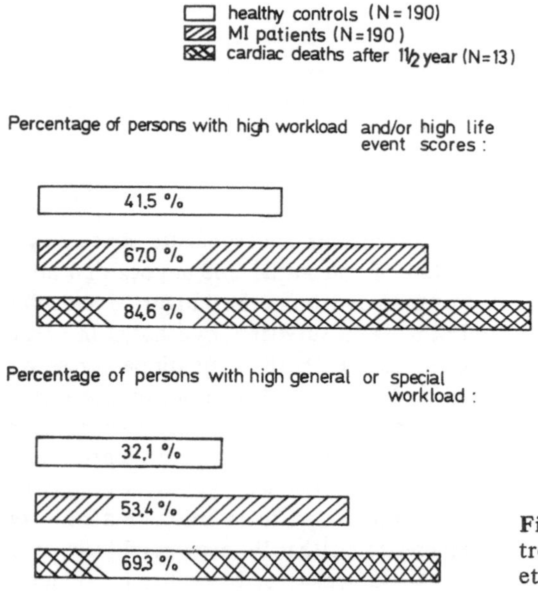

☐ healthy controls (N = 190)
▨ MI patients (N = 190)
▧ cardiac deaths after 1½ year (N = 13)

Percentage of persons with high workload and/or high life event scores :

41,5 %

67,0 %

84,6 %

Percentage of persons with high general or special workload :

32,1 %

53,4 %

69,3 %

Fig. 6. Social risk situations of healthy controls, MI subjects and cardiac deaths (Siegrist et al. 1980)

prospectively to the occurence of CHD has not yet been effectuated to our knowledge" (Kornitzer et al. 1981). This is exactly one of the points where future research has to take off.

References

Birkenhäger WH, Falge HE (1978) Circulating catecholamines and blood pressure. Bunge, Utrecht

Cobb S, Rose M (1973) Hypertension, peptic ulcer and diabetes in air-traffic controllers. JAMA 224:489–492

Dembroski TM, Halhuber MJ (eds) (to be published) Das koronar-gefährdende Verhaltensmuster. Springer, Berlin Heidelberg New York

Epstein FH (1979) Predicting, explaining and preventing coronary heart disease. An epidemiological view. Mod Concepts Cardiovasc Dis 48:2

Folkow B (1975) Vascular changes in hypertension: Review and recent animal studies. In: Berglund C, et al (eds) Pathophysiology and management of arterial hypertension. Lindgren, Mölndal, pp 95–113

Frankenhaeuser M (1979) Psychoneuro-endocrine approaches to the study of emotions as related to stress and coping. In: Howe M, Dienstbier R (eds) Nebraska Symposium on Motivation. University of Nebraska Press, pp 123–161

Frankenhaeuser M (1980) Psychobiological aspects of life-stress. In: Levine S, Ursin H (eds) Coping and health. Plenum

Frankenhaeuser M (to be published) Psycho neuro-endocrine aspects of effort and distress as modified by personal control. In: Sinz R (ed) Proceedings of psycho-physiology. Fischer, Berlin

Galosy RA, Gaebelein CJ (1977) Cardio-vascular adaptation to environmental stress: Its role in the development of hypertension, responsible mechanisms and hypotheses. Biobehav Rev 1:165–175

Ganten D (ed) (1980) Weißbuch Hypertonie. Die Bluthochdruckkrankheit. Wissensstand — Analysen — Konsequenzen. Fischer, Stuttgart, New York

Glass DC (1981) Type A behavior: Mechanisms linking behavior and pathophysiologic processes. In: Siegrist J, Halhuber MJ (eds) Myocardial infarction and psychosocial risks. Springer, Berlin Heidelberg New York, pp 77–89

Henry JP, Stephens P (1977) Stress, health and the social environment. Springer, Berlin Heidelberg New York

Kavoussi N (1973) The relationship between the length of exposure to noise and the incidence of hypertension. Med Lav 64:293

Kornitzer M et al (1981) Work load and coronary heart disease. In: Siegrist J, Halhuber MJ (eds) Myocardial infarction and psychosocial risks. Springer, Berlin Heidelberg New York, pp 18–40

Lown B et al (1977) Neural and psychological mechanisms and the problem of sudden cardiac death. Am J Cardiol 39:890–902

Raab W (1970) Preventive myocardiology. Thomas, Springfield

Selye H (1976) Stress in health and disease. Butterworths, Boston

Siegrist J, Halhuber MJ (eds) (1981) Myocardial infarction and psychosocial risks. Springer, Berlin Heidelberg New York

Siegrist J et al (1980) Soziale Belastungen und Herzinfarkt. Springer, Berlin Heidelberg New York

Suvorov GA et al (1979) Über die Korrelation des Gehörverlustes und neuro-vaskulärer Schädigungen bei Arbeitern in Abhängigkeit vom Lärmniveau (in Russian). Gig Tr Prof Zabol 7:18

Taggart P et al (1971) Endogenous hyperlipidaemia induced by emotional stress of racing drive. Lancet I:363–366

The Role of Protective Factors

F.H. Epstein

The term "risk factor" appeared for the first time in a Framingham publication 20 years ago. The expression "protective factor" hung, as it were, in the air ever since it was debated whether physical activity protects against coronary heart disease. However, it gained wide use only after the inverse relationship between coronary heart disease risk and high-density lipoportein (HDL) was rediscovered around 1975. It may be questioned if the division between risk and protective factors is fortunate. It makes little difference whether one talks about physical *in*activity as a risk factor or physical activity as a protective factor. Similarly, a low low-density lipoprotein (LDL) level is as much of a protective factor as a high HDL level! There ist, nevertheless, a psychological advantage to the term "protective factor" from the preventive point of view since people may be more ready to do something positive to protect their health than something, as they see it, negative (i.e. give up something) to avoid risk.

This brief review will deal with the two "protective factors" mentioned already — physical activity and HDL. Before proceding, let it be remembered that a low level of the major risk factors (serum cholesterol, blood pressure, and smoking) is probably more protective than anything else known or discovered since; the multivariate risk, based on these three risk factors, is six times lower in the fifth of the male population with the lowest score than in the fifth with the highest [1]!

Physical Activity

It has been known since the 1960s and earlier that physically active men have, based on the evidence of nearly all published reports, a lower mortality and morbitidy of coronary heart disease than their less active counterparts [2]. The most recent reports are based on large, prospective studies amongst San Francisco longshoremen [3], Harvard University alumni [4], British civil servants [3], and the Framingham population [6].

All of these studies indicated that physically active men have a lower risk (Table 1). The data are remarkably consistent, the difference in risk between high and low activity level being about three-fold. Critics will say now, as they have been saying for the past 20 or more years, that the difference may be due to pre-selection, constitutionally more healthy men being more likely to become physically active than others, predestined to be sickly. It is imposible to counter this argument short of a randomized intervention study which was shown not to be feasible in the sixties [7]. Certainly, in the four studies shown in Table 1, the advantage of physically active men is largely independent of other risk factors. It is reasonable to conclude that, for all practical purposes, physical activity is protective, unless the great multitude of studies, all pointing in this direction, are subject to the same bias of pre-selection which seems inherently unlikely though not entirely impossible.

Table 1. Physical activity and relative risk of myocardial infarction amongst men

Author	Population		Physical activity High	Inter- mediate	Low
Pfaffenbarger (1977)[a]	Longshoremen	born 1897–1906	1.0	2.9	3.3
		born 1907–1916	1.0	2.5	2.8
Pfaffenbarger (1978)[b]	Harvard University alumni	age 35–44	1.0	–	2.8
		45–54	1.0	–	1.3
		55–64	1.0	–	2.5
		65–74	1.0	–	2.3
Morris (1980)[b]	British civil servants	age 40–65	1.0	← 2.2 →	
Dawber (1980)[c]	Framingham population	age 30–39	1.0	1.0	3.0
		40–49	1.0	1.8	3.1
		50–59	1.0	1.5	2.7

a Data confined to fatal heart attacks; physical activity at work only assessed
b Physical activity at work not included
c All physical activity included

High-Density Lipoprotein

There can be little doubt that CHD risk is less in men with higher HDL concentration in the serum. The evidence comes from epidemiological studies, as well as angiographic and pathological observations. It is not known whether HDL is protective in an active sense, preventing entry of low-density lipoprotein into cells and facilitating their removal, or whether a high HDL level is merely an index of a faster and more effective turnover of very low, intermediate, or low-density lipoproteins, thus preventing their cellular accumulation.

The view is frequently expressed nowadays that total serum cholesterol measurements for assessing CHD risk are passé. This opinion requires critical scrutiny (Fig. 1). The data in this chart are based on the Pooling Project and the so-called "multipliers" of the Framingham study which can be used to assess the protective effect of HDL [8, 9]. The data had to be calculated because there is no published information on CHD risk at various combinations of total and HDL cholesterol levels. It is apparent that CHD risk rises with decreasing level of HDL within all the three ranges of total serum cholesterol (the irregularity for the combination HDL cholesterol 40–49 mg% and total cholesterol below 220 mg% is probably due to the small number of subjects in this group). From the point of view of screening for people at high risk, the question arises how much information is provided by HDL above and beyond the predictive power contained in total cholesterol alone. At total cholesterol levels of 270 mg% or higher, the risk is too high even for that third of this group with the highest HDL, considering that these men carry a risk of 100 per 1000, corresponding to the average population risk which is generally judged to be excessive. Seen in this light, HDL gives no additional information, except for the fact that two-thirds of such men are at particularly high risk and should be motivated even more strongly to improve their lipid pattern. At the other end of the scale, at levels of total cholesterol under 220 mg%, one-third of these men carry an unduly high risk on account of a low HDL level. From

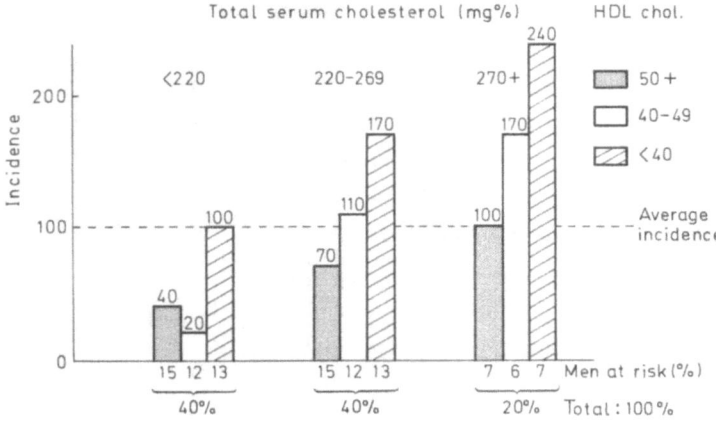

Fig. 1. Incidence of myocardial infarction and sudden death[1] (per 1000 in 10 years; men aged 40–59)

the point of view of individual prevention, it would certainly be desirable to identify these persons specifically. From the point of view of screening a population for high-risk people, however, the question arises whether it is worthwhile taking HDL measurements, in addition to total serum cholesterol, in order to detect only 13% of the entire population of men who might be given a false sense of security on account of their relatively low total serum cholesterol level.

Lastly, what can be done about HDL from the point of view of prevention? The aim will be to keep HDL in relation to LDL high. While LDL rises with age, HDL does not [10]. The first aim, therefore, will be to prevent the rise of LDL with age, primarily by dietary means and weight control. Physical activity is said to raise HDL but there is at least one report which suggests that HDL and LDL both decline during a programme of physical training [11]. Actually, in cross-cultural studies, in contrast to studies within the same country, total serum cholesterol (i.e. LDL) and HDL are positively correlated so that persons with lower total serum cholesterol also have lower levels of HDL [12]. Further research is needed to find the best ways to keep, at the same time, LDL optimally low and HDL optimally high. Amongst other factors affecting HDL, alcohol causes increases while overweight and smoking are associated with lower HDL levels [13].

Conclusions

Risk of coronary heart disease is related to elevated levels of LDL, low levels of HDL, raised blood pressure, smoking, lack of exercise and, in all likelihood, certain patterns of psycho-social stress. For all of these factors, the evidence is strong that they are causally linked to pathogenic mechanisms in the arteries and the myocardium [9]. A strategy of protection against coronary heart disease could be based on keeping these influences within optimal

---

1 Calculated from Pooling Project and Framingham data

ranges throughout life, if there was a will and determination to act and develop corresponding preventive programmes.

References

1 Pooling Project Research Group (1978) Relationship of blood pressure, serum cholesterol, smoking habit, relative weight and ECG abnormalities to incidence of major coronary events: Final report of the Pooling Project. J Chronic Dis 31:201−306
2 Epstein FH (1968) Multiple risk factors and the prediction of coronary heart disease. Bull NY Acad Med 44:916−935
3 Pfaffenbarger RS, Hale WE, Brand RJ, Hyde RT (1977) Work-energy level, personal characteristics, and fatal heart attack: A birth-cohort effect. Am J Epidemiol 105:200−213
4 Pfaffenbarger RS Jr, Wing AL, Hyde RT (1978) Physical activity as an index of heart attack risk in college alumni. Am J Epidemiol 108:161−175
5 Morris JN, Everitt MG, Pollard R, Chave SPW (1980) Vigorous exercise in leisure-time: Protection against coronary heart disease. Lancet II:1207−1210
6 Dawber TR (1980) The Framingham Study: The epidemiology of atherosclerotic disease. Harvard University Press, Cambridge, Mass., London
7 Taylor HL, Buskirk ER, Remington RD (1973) Exercise in controlled trials of the prevention of coronary heart disease. Fed Proc 32:1623−1627
8 Epstein FH (1980) Role of HDL in individuel prediction and community prevention of coronary heart disease. In: Gotto AM Jr, Smith LC, Allen B (eds) Atherosclerosis V. Proceed. of the 5th Int. Symp. on Atherosclerosis. Springer, Berlin Heidelberg New York, pp 484−487
9 Epstein FH (1980) Die Lipidtherorie: epidemiologische Evidenz. Ther Umsch 37:947−953
10 Rifkind BM, Tamir I, Heiss G, Wallace RB, Tyroler HA (1979) Distribution of high density and other lipoproteins in selected LRC Prevalence Study Populations: A brief survey. Lipids 14:105−112
11 Diehm C, Mörl H, Wieland H, Hoffmann G, Tripke A, Oster P, Halhuber MJ, Schettler G (1980) Der Einfluß eines vierwöchigen körperlichen Trainings auf die Serumlipide bei Patienten nach Myokardinfarkt. In: Müller-Wiefel H, Barras J-P, Ehringer H, Krüger M (eds) Mikrozirkulation und Blutrheologie. Witzstrock, Baden-Baden Köln New York
12 Knuiman JT, Hermus RJJ, Hautvast JGAJ (1980) Serum total and high density lipoproteins (HDL) cholesterol concentrations in rural and urban boys from 16 countries. Atherosclerosis 36:529−537
13 Hulley SB (1978) The high density lipoproteins: An epidemiological review. Adv Exp Med Biol 109:295−315

Do the Standard Risk Factors Alter Their Role After the First Myocardial Infarction?

F.H. Epstein and L. Wilhelmsen

There is no a priori reason why the risk factors which help to predict a first event of myocardial infarction should also have value in predicting the risk of recurrence. In all likelihood, predictive power is based on the correlation between the level of risk factors and the degree and progression of coronary atherosclerosis. Patients who survived a myocardial infarction usually have a high degree of arterial disease already and risk factors could only be correlated with the further rate of progression. The extent to which this might be true will be discussed. In this light, it is probable that risk factors would not influence short-term prognosis but possibly gain in importance as time goes on after a first event. There is no question that short-term prognosis and, to a lesser degree, long-term survival are not determined primarily by the amount of myocardial damage and the impairment of cardiac function. It will be apparent that data on the predictiveness of risk factors after myocardial infarction are rather scant.

The Major Risk Factors

Three long-term studies bear in the predictive value of the major risk factors (Table 1). In Framingham [1] and the Göteborg Study (submitted for publication), blood pressure measured after the event is not predictive. This is hardly surprising since blood pressure frequently falls and remains lower after the attack. A significant relation has, however, been demonstrated in the Coronary Drug Project [2]. Data relating the risk factor level before the event to the risk of recurrence have been reported from Framingham only [1, 3]; a significant relationship is noted only for blood pressure. As regards serum cholesterol, measured after the event, a relationship is found in only the Coronary Drug Project [4]. Smoking predicts recurrence both in Göteborg and the Coronary Drug Project but, oddly, there is a negative, though nonsignificant association in Framingham [3]. However, it should be recalled that the risk of recurrence in Framingham men who stop smoking is sharply reduced [5], as it is also in the Göteborg Study [6].
From the evidence, it may be concluded that the influence of the three major risk factors cannot be discounted, but the data are far less unequivocal than in the case of predicting a first attack.

Other Risk Factors

Concerning physical activity and the risk of recurrence, the data from the HIP (Health Insurance Plan) study in New York, published in 1968, remain valid and still stand alone [7]; men who were physically more active clearly had a better prognosis. For diabetes, the risk of recurrence is significantly greater in the presence than in the absence of this condition, except in the period of 3 months to 3 years after myocardial infarction, in the Göteborg

Table 1. Predictive value of risk factors for total mortality after myocardial infarction (MI) amongst men

Study	Blood pressure measured		Serum cholesterol measured		Smoking measured	
	before MI	after MI	before MI	after MI	before MI	after MI
Framingham study	Yes	No	No	No	Yes + (NS)	Yes - (NS)
Göteborg study	—	No	—	No	—	Yes
Coronary drug project	—	Yes	—	Yes	—	Yes

NS: Not significant

Study (submitted for publication). No such relationship exists in the Framingham data, which are, however, based on glucose level rather than the diagnosis of diabetes [3]. Finally, the risk of recurrence in the Western Collaborative Study is greater for type A than for type B men [8].

Summarizing the evidence, there is once again reason to postulate a relationship between risk of disease and risk factors, in this instance physical inactivity, diabetes and emotional behaviour. As regards the preventive value of physical activity, there is furthermore at least one published intervention study which shows a positive result [9].

Conclusion

Existing data suggest that survival after infarction is not entirely determined by the state and function of the myocardium, but that the control of risk factors, even after the event, may have protective value. It must be recognized that any lack of association between a risk factor, e.g. serum cholesterol, and the risk of recurrence by no means *necessarily* means that a reduction in risk factor level might not result in slowing the progress of disease and, therefore, improve prognosis. A recent joint statement, published by the Councils of Arteriosclerosis, Epidemiology and Prevention, and Rehabilitation of the International Society of Cardiology [10] reflects this positive attitude.

It must be kept in mind that observational data obtained after myocardial attack are much more difficult to interpret than those collected prior to the event because the natural course of the disease is modified by a variety of treatment. This problem will become intensified with the growing introduction of more potent drugs, especially beta-blockers and agents affecting platelets and haemostasis, notwithstanding all the controversy surrounding their efficacy. It may well be that valid answers to the questions relating to risk factors and prognosis can only come, at this stage, from controlled intervention studies.

References

1   Kannel WB, Sorlie P, Castelli WP, McGee D (1980) Blood pressure and survival after myocardial infarction — Framingham Study. Am J Cardiol 45:326—331
2   Coronary Drug Project Research Group (1974) Factors influencing long-term prognosis after recovery from myocardial infarction — three years finding of the Coronary Drug Project. J Chronic Dis 27:267—287
3   The Framingham Study (1977) An epidemiological investigation of cardiovascular disease. Section 32: Cardiovascular diseases and death following myocardial infarction and angina pectoris, Framingham Study, 20 years follow-up. U.S. Dept. of Health, Education and Welfare, PHS, NIH, DHEW Publ. No. (NIH) 77—1247
4   Coronary Drug Project Research Group (1978) Natural history of myocardial infarction in the coronary drug project: Long-term prognostic importance of serum lipid levels. Am J Cardiol 42:489—498
5   Gordon T, Kannel W, McGee D, Dawber TR (1974) Death and coronary attacks in men after giving up cigarette smoking. Lancet II:1345—1348
6   Wilhelmsen C, Verdin JA, Elmfeldt D, Tibblin G, Wilhelmsen L (1975) Smoking and myocardial infarction. Lancet I:415—429
7   Frank CW (1968) The course of coronary heart disease: Factors relating to prognosis. Bull NY Acad Med 44:900—915
8   Jenkins CD, Zyzanski SJ, Rosenman RH (1976) Risk of new myocardial infarction in middle-aged men with manifest coronary heart disease. Circulation 53:342—347
9   Kallio V, Hämäläinen H, Hakkila J, Luurila OJ (1979) Reduction in sudden deaths by a multifactorial intervention programme after acute myocardial infarction. Lancet II: 1091—1094
10 Secondary Prevention in Myocardial Infarction Survivors (1980) Joint Recommendations by the International Society and Federation of Cardiology Councils on Atherosclerosis, Epidemiology and Prevention, and Rehabilitation. Heart Beat 3:1—4

Is There a Difference in Risk Factors in the Development of Angina Pectoris and Myocardial Infarction?

M. Kornitzer

Angina pectoris is a subjective symptom with all the fallacies that implies for standardization. Thus various techniques have been used in order to „define" positive cases: most epidemiological studies have used a standardized questionnaire, whereas some have tried to confirm it through a clinical interview with or withour a stress ECG. In clinical series more sophisticated technique are used, like radionuclide investigations and, of course, coronary angiography.

The pathogenesis of angina pectoris has been updated with the reintroduction of an old concept, that of coronary spasm, which can now be visualized during an angiographic procedure, using ergonovine.

In fact besides coronary spasm and atherosclerosis of the large vessels, angina pectoris has been observed in relation with pathological changes of small arteries and with a shift in the oxyhemoglobin dissociation curve, mainly in smokers. Mixed mechanisms are probably involved in variant or Prinzmetal angina (Fig. 1).

The Framingham study has shown that the sex difference for the incidence of the more lethal forms of CHD, i.e., sudden death (SD) and myocardial infarction (MI), is greater than that observed for angina pectoris. This observation is rather puzzling in the light of the important differences in coronary artery stenosis found at autopsy, as shown in Fig. 2, adapted from Diamond and Forrester [2]. These authors calculated probabilities of CHD according to Bayes' theorem in relation with nonanginal chest pain, atypical or typical angina (Table 1).

For nonanginal chest pain, the male/female ratio is over 2 till the age of 59; for atypical angina the ratio is still 1.82 for the age group 50—59, whereas for typical angina the ratio is 1.58 for the age group 40—49, dropping to 1.16 in the age group 50—59. Thus the pretest likelihood of CAD is generally speaking higher in males than females; adding a stress ECG, the subsequent likelihood of CAD is still higher in males. I adapted Figs. 3—5 from Diamond and Forrester [2]. In each case, the lower of the two lines represents the equality equation for males and females. For nonanginal chest pain the post-test likelihood of CAD is systematically higher in males, the regression equation being almost equidistant for the whole set of probabilities: the correlation coefficient is 0.917 and the ratio M/F is over 1, independently of age or level of ST depression (Fig. 3). The same is true for atypical angina, but there, the lines are convergent, meaning that for important (2 mm or more) ST depressions, the post-test likelihoods of CAD for males and females are not very different (Fig. 4).

For typical angina, the post-test likelihood is almost identical for males and females, at least in the higher probability zone (Fig. 5).

In summary, we can reconcile the important sexual differences in pathological findings with the Framingham observation in the light of the concept of coronary spasm, which should be more prevalent in females than males, a hypothesis which has still to be tested.

I would like to turn now to the other coronary risk factors. We initiated 15 years ago prospective studies in two cohorts of bank clerks and will report here results after a follow-up of 10 years, for the two cohorts combined [4]. For serum cholesterol we observed a gradient,

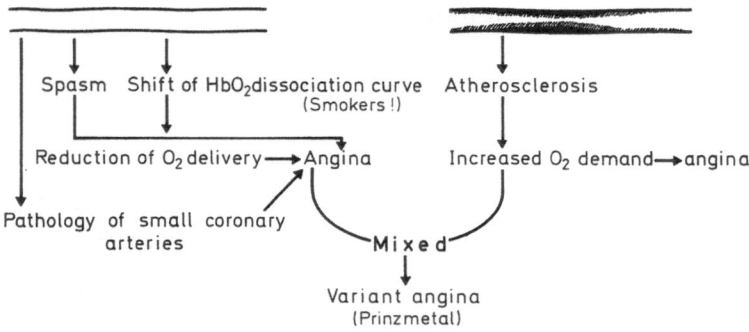

Fig. 1. Pathogenetic pathways of angina pectoris

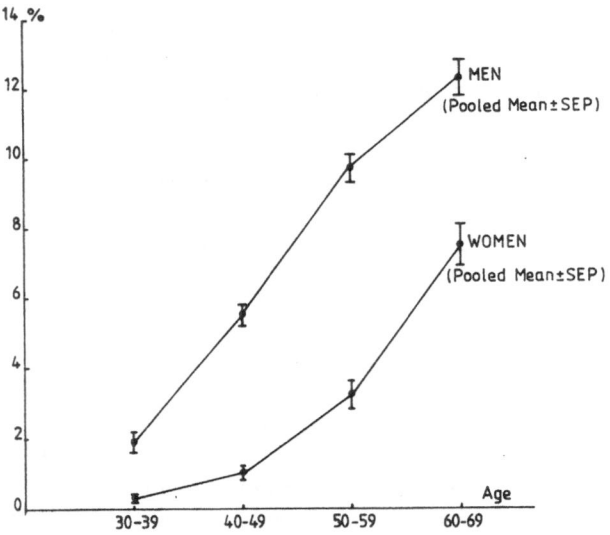

Fig. 2. Prevalence of coronary artery stenosis combining different studies. Adapted from Diamond and Forrester [2]

but the slope for MI and SD is steeper than the one observed for angina pectoris (Fig. 6). Serum cholesterol has been found to be a strong a predictor of angina pectoris as of myocardial infarction in several prospective studies [1, 3, 6].

In our study, systolic blood pressure predicted the risk of MI and SD whereas no systematic relation with the incidence of angina pectoris is observed, although the highest incidence appeared in subjects with baseline blood pressures of 160 mmHg or over (Fig. 7). The same was true for the diastolic blood pressure (Fig. 8).

Whereas the blood pressure level was a good predictor of angina pectoris in the Framingham study [6], this has not been observed in other prospective studies [1, 3].

Table 1. Pretest likelihood of CAD in symptomatic patients according to age and sex

Age	Nonanginal chest pain			Atypical angina			Typical angina		
	Male %	Female %	Ratio M/F	Male %	Female %	Ratio M/F	Male %	Female %	Ratio M/F
30–39	5.2	0.8	6.50	21.8	4.2	5.19	69.7	25.8	2.70
40–49	14.1	2.8	5.04	46.1	13.3	3.47	87.3	55.2	1.58
50–59	21.5	8.4	2.56	58.9	32.4	1.82	92.0	79.4	1.16
60–69	28.1	18.6	1.51	67.1	54.4	1.23	94.3	90.6	1.04

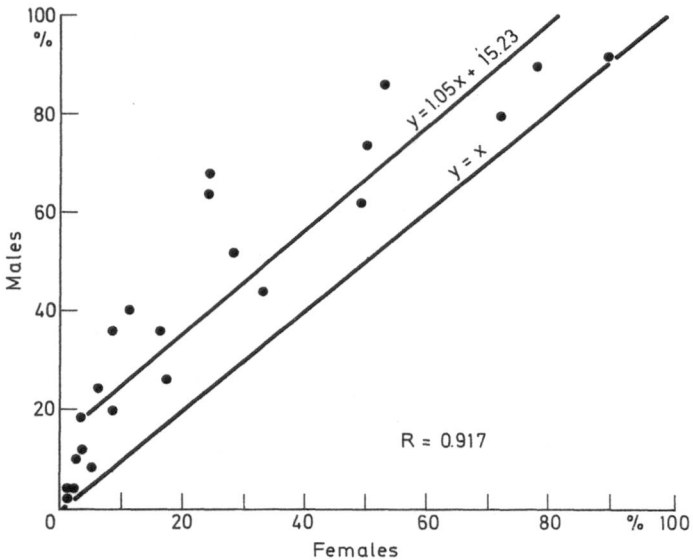

Fig. 3. Post-test likelihood of CAD in males and females complaining of chest pain. Adapted from Diamond and Forrester [2]

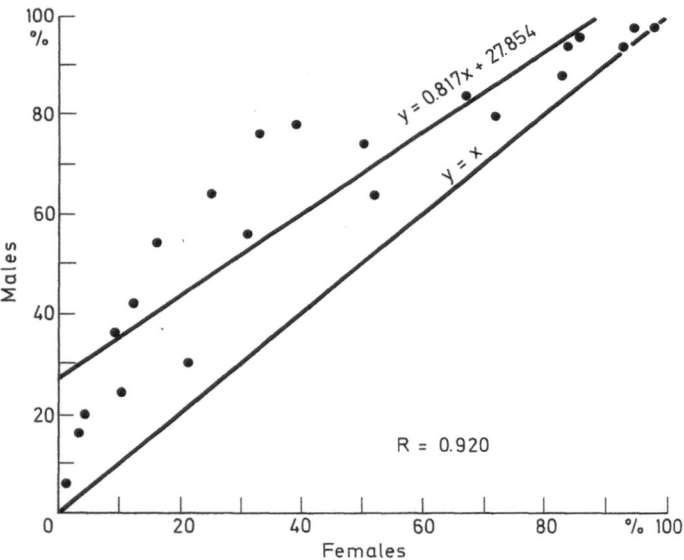

Fig. 4. Post-test likelihood of CAD in males and females complaining of "atypical" angina. Adapted from Diamond and Forrester [2]

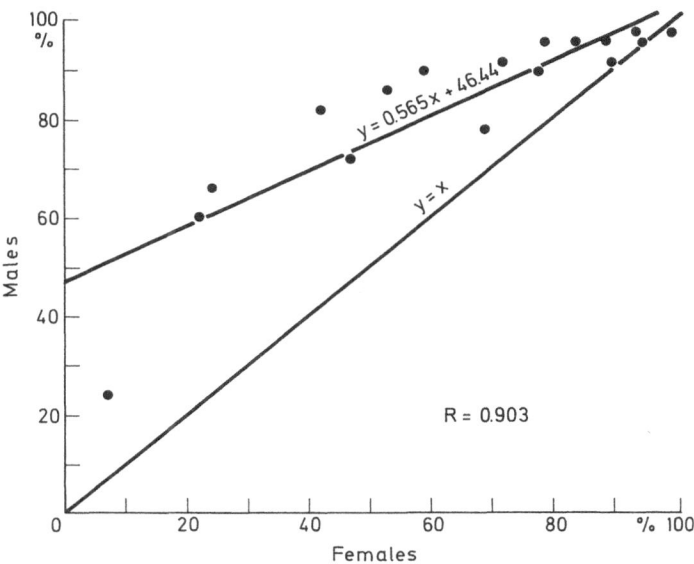

Fig. 5. Post-test likelihood of CAD in males and females complaining of typical angina. Adapted from Diamond and Forrester [2]

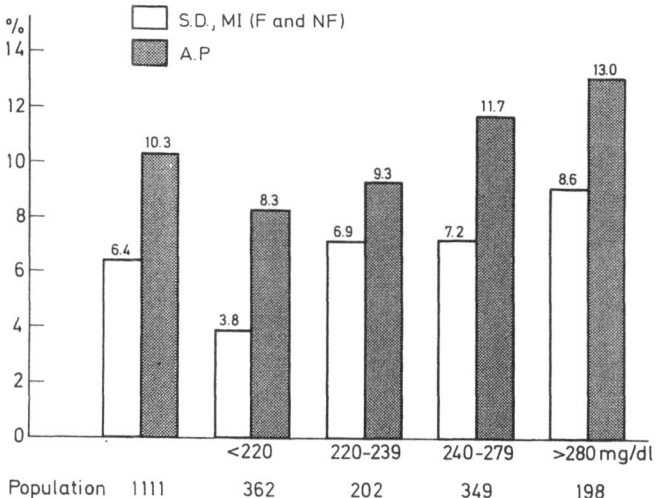

Fig. 6. Ten-year incidence of CAD in 1111 middle-aged Belgian males free of CAD at entry in relation to baseline serum cholesterol

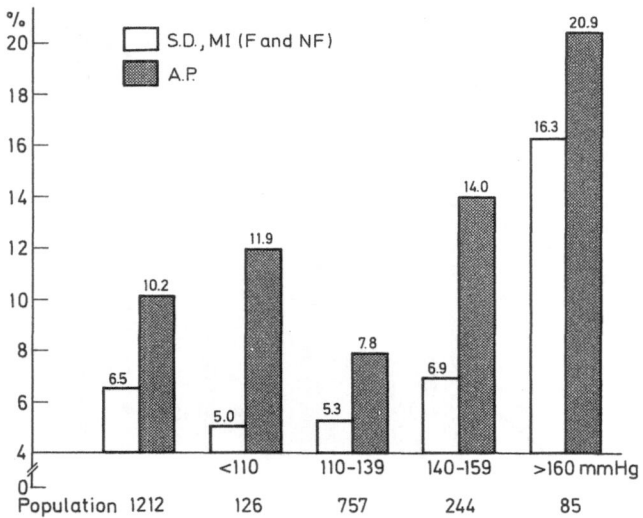

Fig. 7. Ten-year incidence of CAD in 1212 middle-aged Belgian males free of CAD at entry in relation to baseline systolic blood pressure

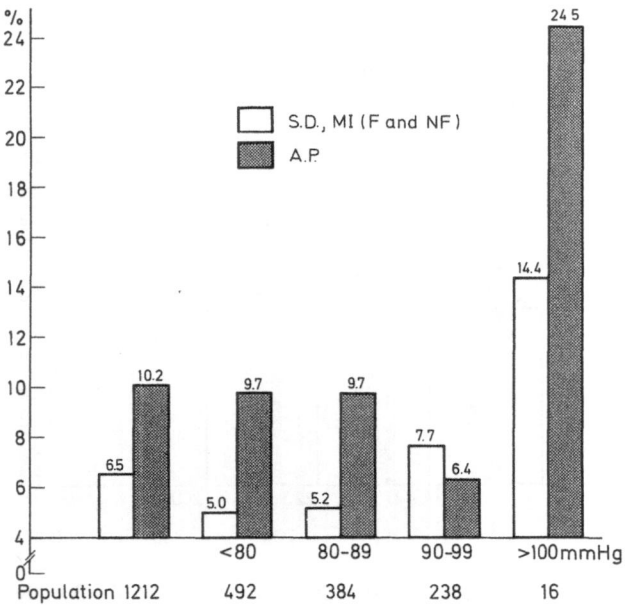

Fig. 8. Ten-year incidence of CAD in 1212 middle-aged Belgian males free of CAD at entry in relation to baseline diastolic blood pressure

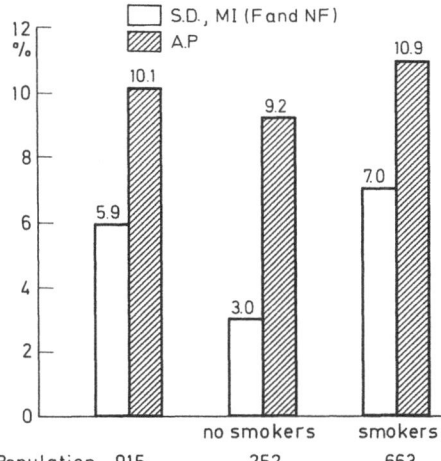

Fig. 9. Ten-year incidence of CAD in 915 middle-aged Belgian males according to baseline smoking habits

In our study, the risk of MI and SD is twice as high in cigarette smokers as in life-long non-smokers whereas a trivial difference was observed for angina pectoris (Fig. 9), and this was indeed the fact in most of the studies reviewed.

As for physical activity, Paffenbarger et al. [5] related the risk of angina pectoris in college alumni, according to a physical activity index: they reported a relative risk of 1.91 for angina pectoris, for an index < 2000 kcal/week/ ⩾ 2000 kcal/week.

In summary, I feel that the relation of the classical coronary risk factors with angina pectoris is not as clear-cut as that observed for myocardial infarction and sudden death, apart from serum cholesterol level. Different pathogenetic mechanisms behind the same symptom could be an explanation.

References

1 Chapman JM, Coulson AH, Clark VA, Borun ER (1971) The differential effect of serum cholesterol, blood pressure and weight on the incidence of myocardial infarction and angina pectoris. J Chronic Dis 23:631−645

2 Diamond GA, Forrester JS (1979) Analysis of probability as an aid in the clinical diagnosis of coronary-artery disease. N Engl J Med 24:1350−1358

3 Holme I, Helgeland A, Hjermann I, Leren P, Lund-Larsen PG (1980) Four and two-thirds years incidence of coronary heart disease in middle-aged men: The Oslo Study. Am J Epidemiol 112:149−160

4 Kornitzer M, Dramaix M, Gheyssens H (1979) Incidence of ischemic heart diseases in two Belgian cochorts followed during 10 yr. Eur J Cardiol 9/6:455−472

5 Pfaffenbarger RS Jr, Wing AL, Hyde RT (1978) Physical activity as an index of heart attack risk in college alumni. Am J Epidemiol 108:161−175

6 The Framingham Study (1974) An epidemiological investigation of cardiovascular disease (Section 30): Some characteristics related to the incidence of cardiovascular disease and death: Framingham Study, 18-year follow-up. U.S. Govt. Printing Office, DHEW Publ. No(NIH) 74−599. Washington D.C.

The Reasons for Recommending Physical Training as a Preventive Measure Following Myocardial Infarction

W. Hollmann

The Reasons for Recommending Physical Training as Preventive Measure in Healthy Persons. Before the influence and the importance of physical training on a patient with myocardial infarction is discussed, the effect of physical training on healthy persons will be explained in a few sentences. For this purpose we must make a distinction between the five main types of motor strain: coordination, flexibility, strength, speed, and endurance. Only endurance training has the required influence on the cardiopulmonary system and the metabolism. For instance, it is not possible to achieve important preventive training stimuli through exercising flexibility or static or dynamic strength training. In healthy persons we trained large groups of muscles through various forms of strength training (Fig. 1). On average, total strength increased by 36%. The maximum oxygen uptake, the major criterion of cardiopulmonary capacity, remained within the scattering range of the original value.

By improving basic speed and speed endurance it is not possible to achieve adaptations of the heart that are valuable from the point of view of prevention. This form of training produces a high lactate level with a low pH value within the muscle, which is undesirable for the cardiopulmonary system.

This leaves us with *endurance* and *coordination*. Only general aerobic endurance, as it is known, is of clinical importance. A suitable *minimum training program* must meet the following requirements:

1. It must involve dynamic work done by large groups of muscles (e.g., running, cycling, swimming, long-distance skiing etc.);
2. The work should be performed continuously for at least 10 min every day. The optimum duration appears to be about 30–40 min a day, repeated three–four times weekly.
3. The work intensity should be high enough to produce a heart rate of 130/min in healthy males and females below the age of 50. In the case of healthy persons who are older than 50, the following general rule can be applied: 180 minus age in years should be the minimum heart rate in training.

This form of training causes *peripheral adaptations* in two categories: metabolic and haemodynamic. Metabolic adaptations consist in an increase in the number and size of the mitochondria in the trained skeletal muscle (Fig. 2), an increase in the activity of aerobic enzymes (Fig. 3), and an increase in the myoglobin and the glycogen content.

Peripheral haemodynamic adaptations consist in an improved capillarization of the muscle (Fig. 4).

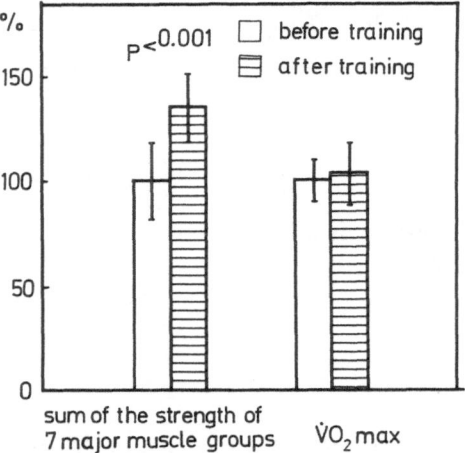

Fig. 1. Increase in strength of big muscle groups after strength training *(left side)*, while the $\dot{V}O_2$ max is nearly unchanged *(right side)*

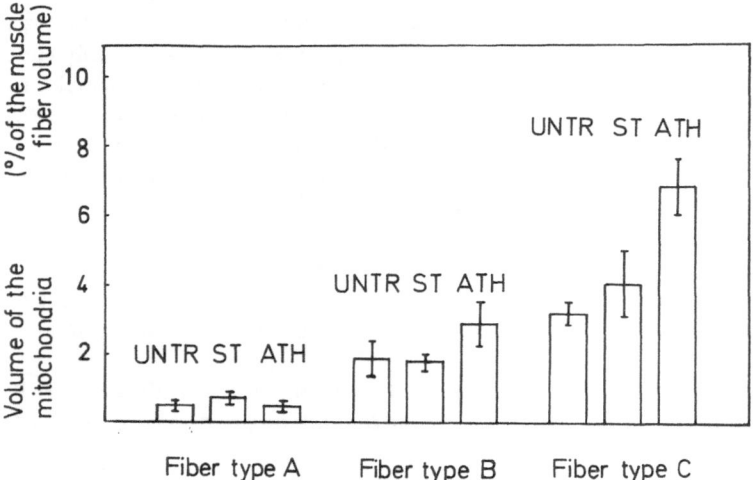

Fig. 2. Percentage of mitochondrial volume in the three fiber types in normal persons (I), sports students (II), and endurance trained persons (III) [14]

As a *result* of peripheral adaptation, the local aerobic performance capacity increases and the peripheral sympathetic stimulation is reduced (Figs. 5, 6).

The *central adaptation* consist of: A reduction in the heart rate at rest and at any given level of work, and, in some cases, a drop in the systolic blood pressure during a given workload; a prolongation of diastole; a reduction in the peripheral resistance; a reduction in the release of catecholamines at given levels of work (Figs. 7–10).

All these mechanisms lead to a reduction in the oxygen requirements within the myocardium. *This factor is the most important one for preventive cardiology.* The prolongation of diastole extends the most important phase in which blood is supplied to the myocardium.

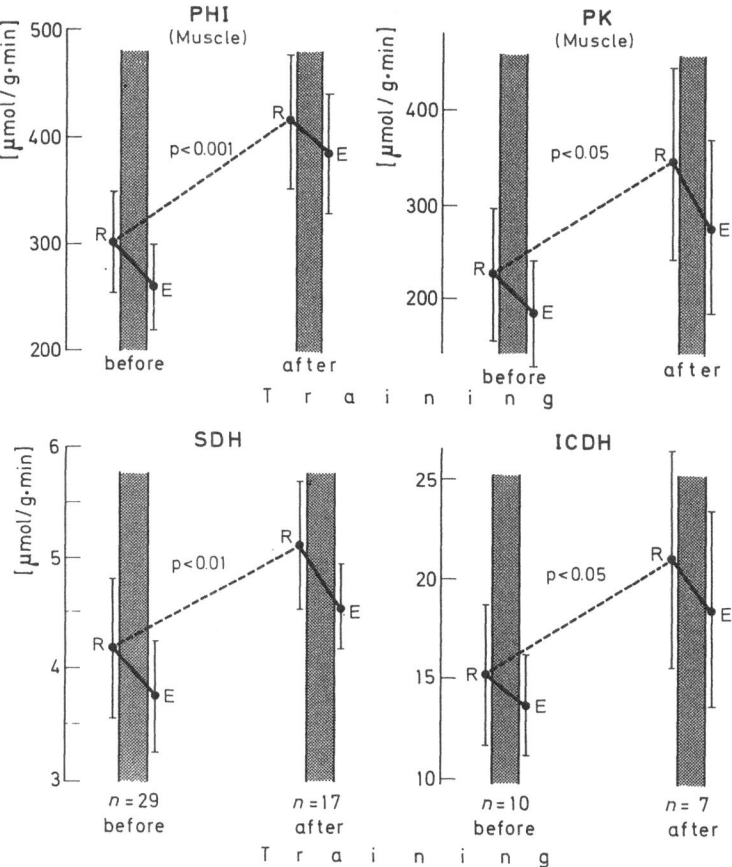

Fig. 3. Activities of anaerobic and aerobic enzymes in the m. vastus lateralis before and after a 10-week endurance training in elderly persons (55—70 years of age) [9]

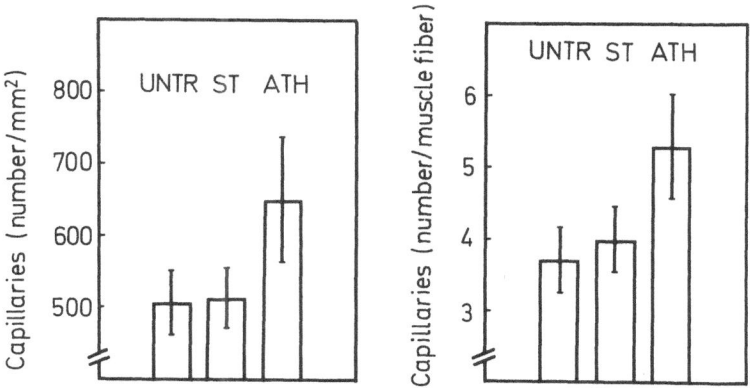

Fig. 4. Number of capillaries per mm^2 and number of capillaries per muscle fibre in m. vastus lateralis in normal persons (I), sport students (II), and endurance trained persons (III) [14]

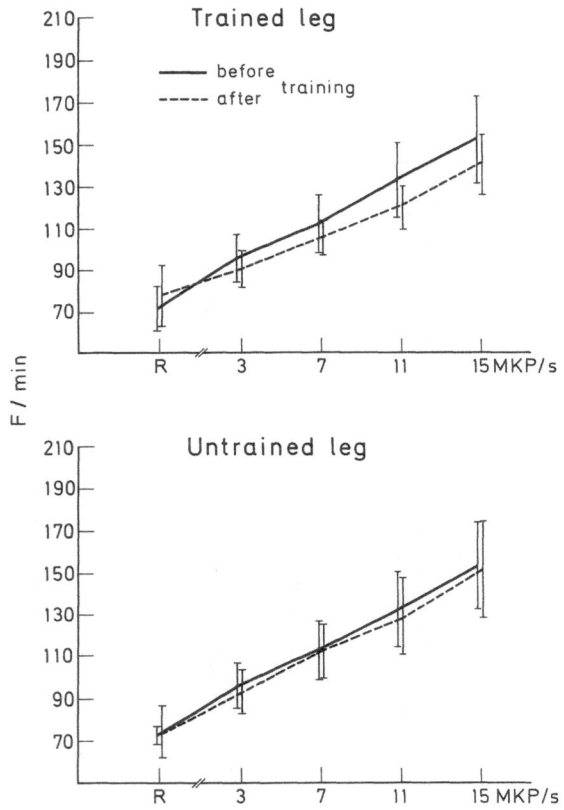

Fig. 5. The heart rate during one-legged-work on the bicycle ergometer before and after an endurance training with one leg (Hollman et al., unpublished work)

The Effect of a Lack of Movement. A *lack of movement* has the opposite effect to endurance training. It is most extreme after prolonged bedrest. In healthy persons who had spent 9 days resting in bed (Fig. 11) we found a reduction in the maximum oxygen uptake of 21% while the radiologically determined heart volume dropped by 10%; the heart rate, respiration volume, and the production of lactic acid increased very intensely for a given work load. Miller and co-workers (Fig. 12) showed, in the same case, an increase of 22% in the mean heart rate at rest, as a result of 14 days bedrest. The oxygen requirement of the myocardium, however, is determined mainly by wall tension, heart rate, and contractility. Clinically it can be characterized by the product of the heart rate and blood pressure. A stay in bed thus results in *an increased* oxygen demand of the heart for any workload.

The Effects of Endurance Training on the Infarction Patient. Which one of the positive effects of endurance training mentioned already can be called upon for use in patients with myocardial infarction? The answer to this question is determined primarily by the maximum tolerable work load of each individual person. *"Maximum tolerable work load"* we call the highest level of physical effort for a given quality of work that can be attained

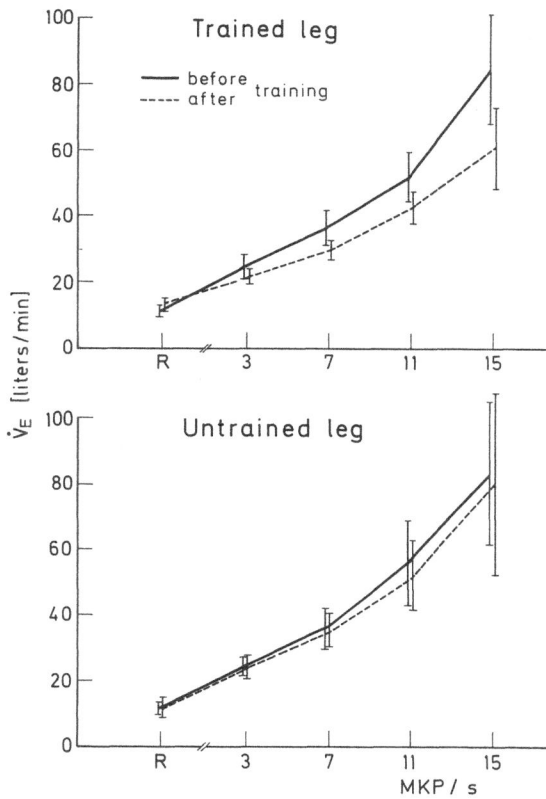

Fig. 6. The ventilation during increasing one-legged work on the bicycle ergometer before and after an endurance training. Significant differences are to be observed only during work with the trained leg, not with the untrained one (Hollmann et al., unpublished work)

without risk. Performance capacity, on the other hand, refers to the maximum performance that can be achieved for a given quality of work. Under normal environmental conditions, for healthy persons below the age of 30, maximum tolerable work load and performance capacity are identical. In the case of coronary patients, however, we must make a careful distinction between the two terms. If the maximum tolerable work load in training permits a work intensity level that enables persons below the age of 60 to attain a heart rate of 120/min and more, then the above-mentioned adaptation mechanisms can be expected to occur. For coronary patients over the age of 60, a heart rate of about 110/min can be regarded as sufficient for this purpose. In these cases it may be expected that an existing disproportion between oxygen supply and oxygen demand in the myocardium will be raised to a higher level of work, thus raising the maximum tolerable work load and creating a zone of relative protection.

If the maximum tolerable work load of the patient is less than 30% of the average normal performance capacity no significant morphological adaptations can be expected to occur. At the same time, in these cases an improvement in the quality of the patient's co-ordination (Fig. 13) can be achieved which causes, in the case of persons unaccustomed to movement, a de-

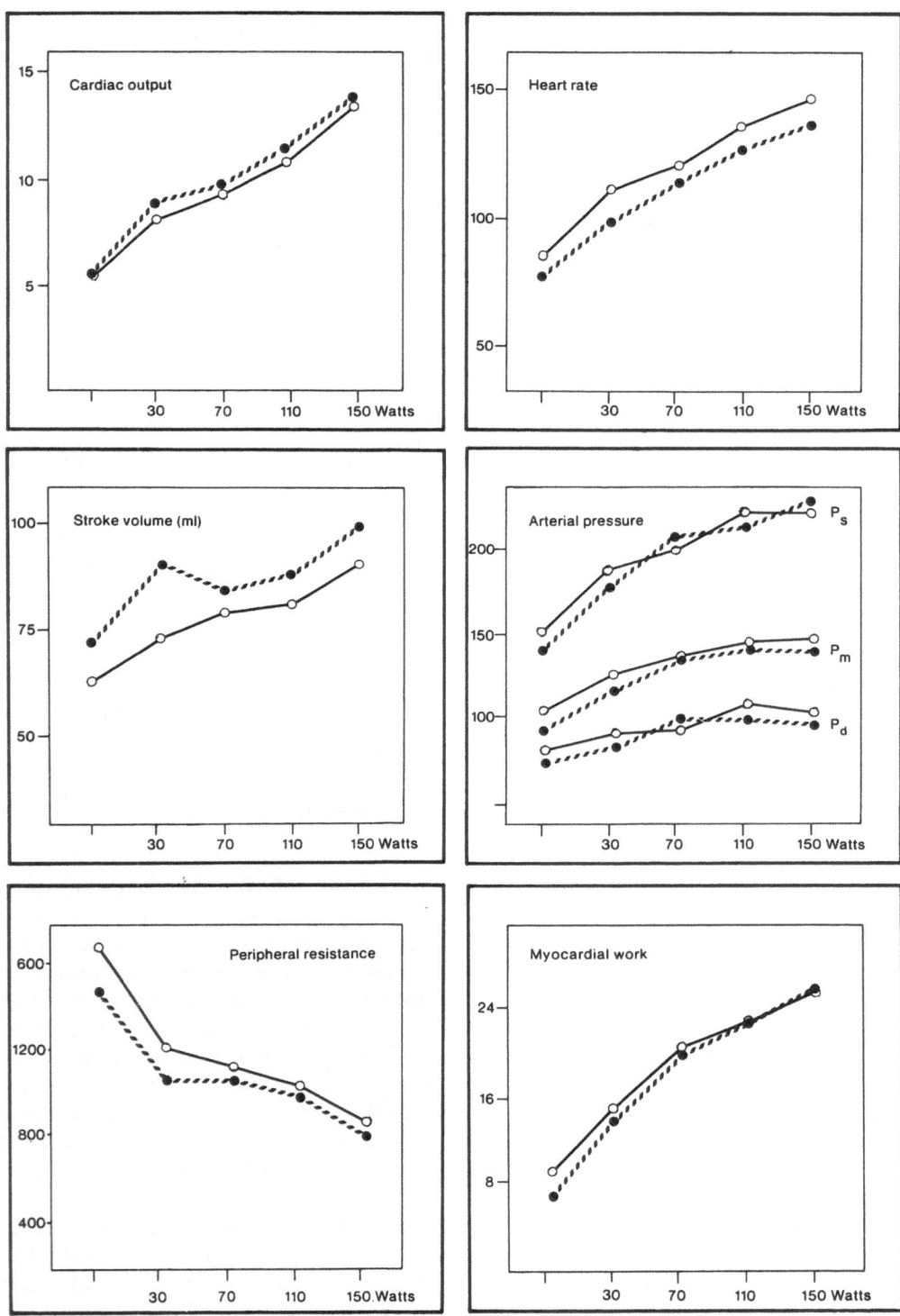

Fig. 7. Haemodynamic parameters before and after a 10-week period of endurance training of elderly male persons (cardiogreen method) [13]

◀——————————————————————————————————

crease in the oxygen requirement for a given work load by at least 10%–15%. This results in a decreased burden on the heart at an unchanged physical performance of the skeletal muscles. Consequently, from a clinical point of view, this aspect is also of value.

In conclusion endurance training prevents the development of an imbalance between oxygen demand and oxygen supply of the myocardium. This might cause a relative protection against anginal attacks. This is supported by a reduced adhesiveness and aggregability of the platelets [1], and an increased fibrinolytic activity [2]. For a given work load the pH value is higher, resulting in better fluid properties of the red cells.

After a training period of 1 year we observed in most infarction patients a significant improvement of the aerobic performance capacity (Fig. 14), a better quality of coordination, an augmented flexibility (Fig. 15), and an enlarged muscle strength (Fig. 16). On the other hand, we also had a small number of patients in our training groups who showed no progress, and in some cases actually showed deterioration.

In recent investigations — together with Feinendegen et al. in the German Nuclear Research Center Jülich — we observed an alteration of metabolic processes in the myocardium of patients with myocardial infarction. They refer in the first study to eight male persons before

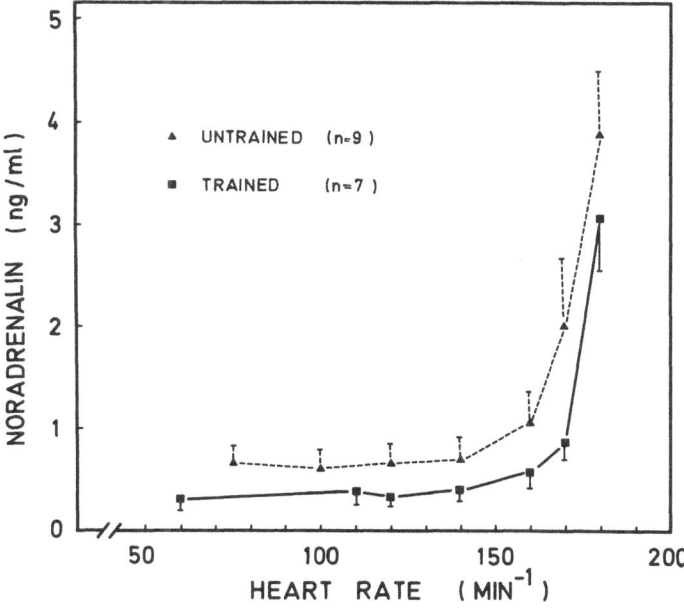

Fig. 8. The norepinephrine level during increasing work on the bicycle ergometer in untrained and endurance-trained persons during identical heart rates. A significant difference is to be seen in spite of the fact that the endurance-trained persons attain higher work loads with any given pulse rate [6]

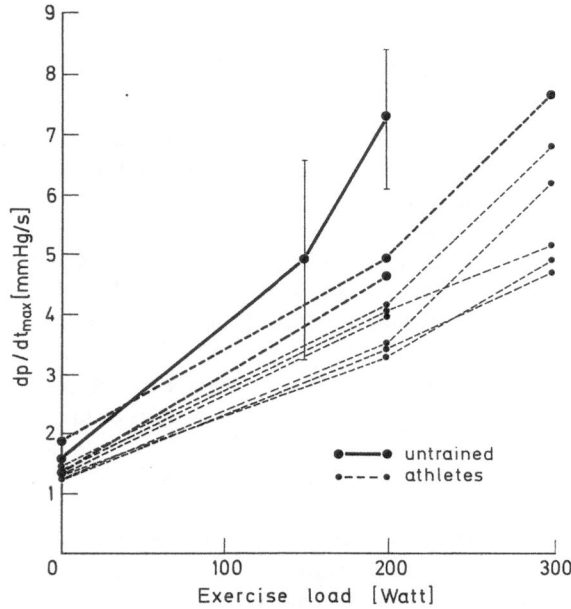

Fig. 9. dp/dt$_{max}$ at rest and during work in endurance-trained persons. The *thick dotted lines* represent the normal area. Endurance training reduced the contractility at a given work load [11]

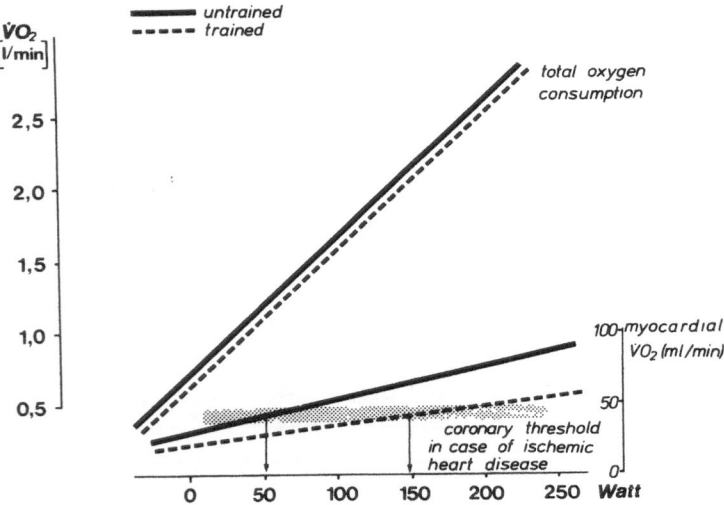

Fig. 10. Schematic representation of the importance of endurance trained for avoiding a disproportion between oxygen requirement and oxygen supply if degenerative coronary alterations exist

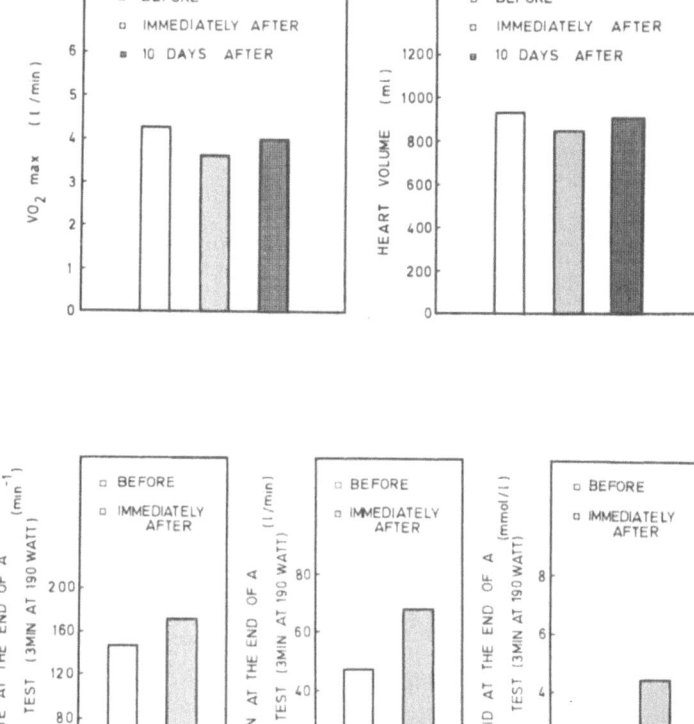

Fig. 11. Maximal oxygen uptake and heart volume after a bedrest of 9 days. Increased pulse rate, ventilation, and lactate during a given work level of 190 watt after the bedrest [4]

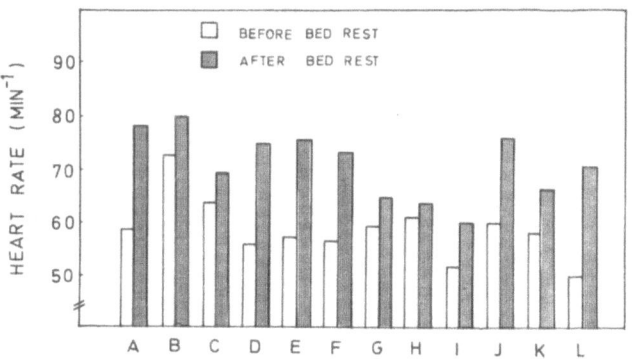

Fig. 12. Average resting heart rates in horizontal position before and after a longer bedrest [10]

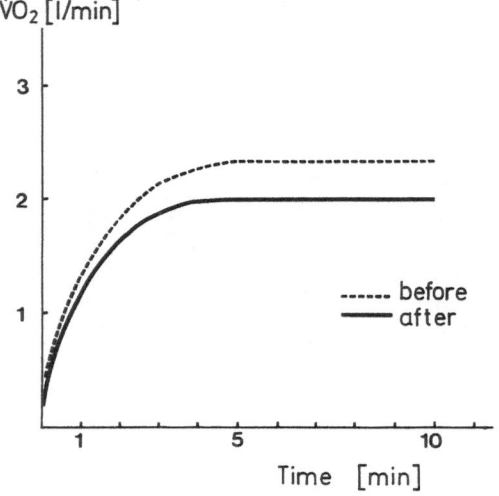

Fig. 13. Reduction of the O_2 requirement for a given running speed on the treadmill after 3 weeks of exercise with a low running velocity [5]

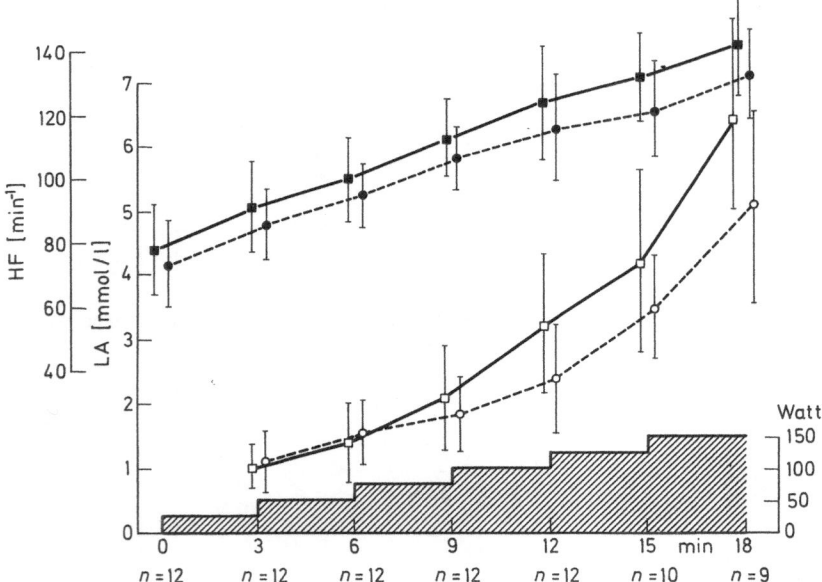

Fig. 14. Reduction in the pulse rate and the lactate level in coronary patients after 1 year of training within a coronary patient group [13]

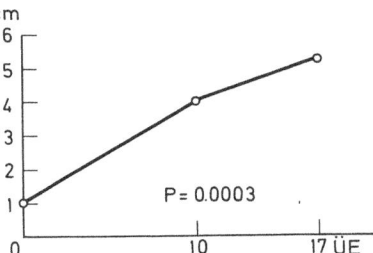

Fig. 15. Improvement of the flexibility in the fingerground test

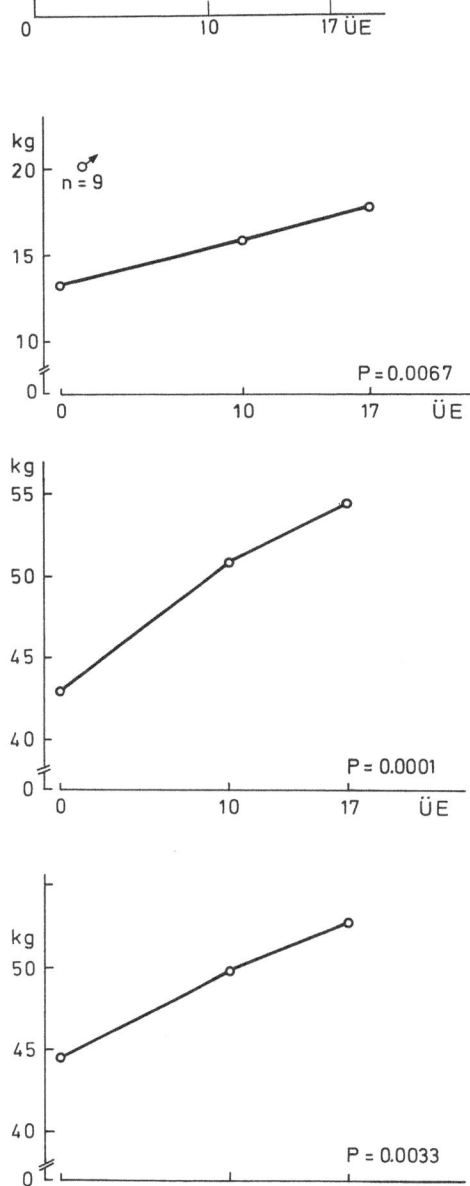

Fig. 16. Improvement of the muscle strength (m. biceps, m. quadriceps, during bending and stretching; n = 87)

and after a physical training period of 12 months. All the patients were given 2.5 mCi I −
123 − HA, followed by 1 mCi 30 min later as an internal standard for correcting the cata-
bolically released iodine. Prior to training, six patients showed a reduction in the total and
segmental rates of elimination: T 1/2 total heart 42−72 min, peri-infarction areas 60−90 min
vs 30 ± 5 min for control. Two patients had normal T 1/2 for the total heart but a prolonged
T 1/2 for the peri-infarction areas (Table 1).

After 12 months training five of the six first mentioned patients revealed a significant improvement in both the overall and the segmental values. The other two patients revealed
only isolated changes in myocardial regions as did five untrained infarction patients with
comparable findings.

It remained an open question to what extent these results indicate an improvement in the
supply of blood to the heart as a result of training. An alternative explanation is that of
intramyocardial, biochemical adaptations with higher oxygen utilization.

At any rate, though, these investigations must be regarded as an initial indication that
physical training may not only influence the skeletal muscles but apparently also affects the
heart directly.

*The Importance of Physical Training for the Reduction of Internal and External Risk Fac-
tors.* Endurance training augments the HDL cholesterol. This is said to give some protection
against the development of degenerative alterations in the arterial wall. There are some other
factors within lipoprotein metabolism which are influenced by endurance training and may
have some importance as a protective factor (Fig. 17).

External risk factors, such as smoking, emotional distress, and also the quantity of nutrition,
can be influenced by physical training. This aspect should not be underestimated in the
case of postinfarction patients.

The increase in physical performance capacity enables people to cope with the problems of
everyday life more easily. This, in return, increases their self-confidence. There is not doubt
that a person's zest for life can be increased in this way and through the social aspect of
contact in the group. In many cases this mental effect of training carried out by postinfarction patients is of immense importance. Physical training is often the first element that makes
life seem worth living again.

Table 1. Elimination half-times in patients with myocardial infarction before (b) and after (a)
rehabilitation training

Patient	Total b	Heart a	Anteroseptal b	a	Segments Inferior b	a	Lateral b	Posterior a
1	30	31	23	24	33	43	38.2	36.4
2	30	29.3	22.8	19.5	37	37.3	37.5	48.6
3	72	38	40.5	25.5	124	59	174	60
4	64	46	71.5	52	56	51	57.5	41.5
5	72	25	43.5	21	92	28	118	26
6	50	31	39.5	23	70	37	57	35
7	42	34	46.5	36.5	34	30	39	29.5
8	65	78	51.8	64	57	56	94	93

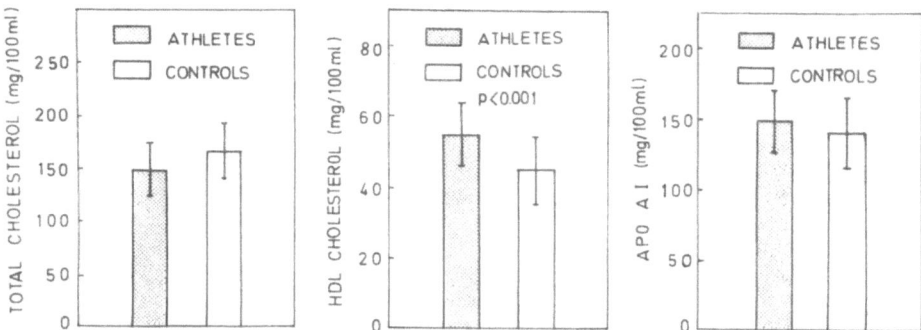

Fig. 17. Total cholesterol, HDL-cholesterol and APO AI in normal persons and endurance-trained athletes [2]

At present it is not possible to say whether or not physical training has a favorable influence on the incidence of reinfarction. Too few studies have been made to allow a conclusive assessment.

To sum up it can be said that, in postinfarction patients, physical training can lead to morphological and functional adaptations which can be considered valuable both from s subjective and also from a physiologic and clinical point of view. Further investigations are necessary, in particular to clarify details of the myocardial adaptations and the question of any influence on the incidence of re-infarction. But even without these findings it can be stated today that, for appropriate patients, physical training can be regarded as an essential part of medical management.

References

1 Broustet JP, Boisseau M, Bouloumie J, Emerau JP, Series E, Bricaod H (1978) The effects of acute exercise and physical training on platelet function in patients with coronary artery disease. Cardic Rehab 9, 2:28

2 Dufaux B, Liesen H, Rost R, Heck H, Hollmann W (1979) Über den Einfluß eines Ausdauertrainings auf die Serum-Lipoproteine unter besonderer Berücksichtigung der Alpha-Lipoproteine (HDL) bei jungen und älteren Personen. Dtsch Z Sportmed 30:123

3 Hollmann W (1959) Der Arbeits- und Trainingseinfluß auf Kreislauf und Atmung. Steinkopff, Darmstadt

4 Hollmann W (1965) Körperliches Training als Prävention von Herz-Kreislaufkrankheiten. Hippokrates, Stuttgart

5 Hollmann W, Hettinger T (1980) Sportmedizin — Arbeits- und Trainingsgrundlagen, 2nd edn., Schattauer, Stuttgart New York

6 Keul J, Huber G, Burmeister P, Steinhilber S, Spielberger B, Zöllner G (1979) Auswirkungen des Autofahrens auf Herztätigkeit und Stoffwechsel. Fortschr Med 97:2172

7 Lagerström D (1978) Das Training mit Infarktpatienten als neuer Aufgabenbereich für den Sportlehrer. Therapiewoche 28:5385

8 Lagerström et al. (1980)

9 Liesen H, Heikinen E, Suominen H, Michel D, Hollmann W (1975) Der Effekt eines 12-wöchigen Ausdauertrainings auf die Leistungsfähigkeit und den Muskelstoffwechsel bei untrainierten Männern des 6. und 7. Lebensjahrzehnts. Sportarzt Sportmed 2:26

10 Miller PB, Johnson RL, Lamb LE (1964) Effects of four weeks of absolute bed rest on circulatory functions in man. Aerospace Med 35:1194

11 Roskamm H (1972) Die Funktion des physiologisch hypertrophierten Myokards. Verh Dtsch Ges Kreislaufforsch 38:77

12 Rost R, Dreisbach W (1975) Zur wissenschaftlichen Begründung körperlichen Trainings als Mittel der Prävention und Rehabilitation bei älteren Menschen. II: Veränderungen im Bereich der zentralen Hämodynamik durch körperliches Training. Sportarzt 2:26

13 Rost R (1979) Kreislaufreaktion und -adaptation unter körperlicher Belastung. Osang, Bonn

14 Schön FA, Hollmann W, Liesen H, Waterloh E (1978) Elektronenmikroskopische Befunde am M. vastus lateralis von Untrainierten und Marathonläufern sowie ihre Beziehung zur relativen maximalen Sauerstoffaufnahme und Laktatproduktion. In: Nowaeki PE, Böhmer D (eds) 26. Deutscher Sportärztekongreß Bad Nauheim. Thieme, Stuttgart New York 1980

15 Williams RS, Logue GL, Barton T, Stead NW, Wallace AG, Pizzo SV (1980) Physical conditioning augments the fibrinolytic response to venous occlusion in healthy adults. N Engl J Med 302:987

Evidence to Date for the Beneficial Effect of Exercise Following Myocardial Infarction

T. Kavanagh

Introduction

There is ample evidence that a post-coronary rehabilitation programme which contains an exercise component is very effective in relieving depression, increasing self-confidence and improving fitness levels [1, 2, 3, 4]. Indeed, there are many who feel that these assets are ample justification in themselves for the proliferation of such programmes [5, 6].

Nevertheless, there still remains the question of prognosis. Does an exercise programme reduce recurrence rates? Obviously the answer can only be sought by means of a clinical trial, either non-randomized or randomized. While experience with the former has suggested that exercise is effective in reducing fatal and non-fatal recurrences [7, 8, 9, 10, 11, 12, 13, 14], one must view such favourable conclusions with caution. The prime objection to the non-randomized study is that the exercisers may be preselected, and thus have a more favourable outlook than the group with which they are compared. Alternatively, bias may be apparent in the non-exercise group who have variously consisted of "drop-outs" from the programme, or those who have refused to exercise (Table 1).

In recent years, to surmount the criticism of preselection, the emphasis has shifted to the so-called randomized controlled trial. Ideally this should provide a valid conclusion as to the efficacy or otherwise of a specific treatment, i.e. a conclusion supported by the weight of statistical analysis. Unfortunately, in my view, the limitations of the randomized trial are all too often not fully appreciated. One can, for instance, miss the positive effect of the proposed treatment and incorrectly conclude that it does not confer any benefit (so-called false positive or beta error) or, alternatively, falsely conclude that the treatment is beneficial (false negative or alpha error); such errors are usually the result of a number of flaws inherent in the original protocol. I propose to cover these briefly, and then illustrate them by reference to the major randomized control studies into the effects of exercise on post-myocardial infarction prognosis which have been carried out to date.

Randomized Trials

Sample Size

The size of the sample under study should be large enough to ensure the detection of a treatment effect, with an acceptably low error rate. The smaller the anticipated final difference between the treated and the control group, and the lower the error rate permitted, the larger the number involved have to be. For example, to detect an end-point difference of 25% instead of 50% between the two groups on a study could require a quadrupling of the sample size. To reduce the possibility of alpha or beta error by 5% can increase the sample size by about 20%.

Table 1. Results of non-randomized trials

	Exercisers Fatal recurrence (%)	Non-fatal recurrence (%)	Controls Fatal recurrence (%)	Non-fatal recurrence (%)	Type of control	Duration (years)
Gottheiner [8] (1968)	0.7	–	2.4	–	Sedentary post-MI	5
Brunner [10] (1968)	3.1	9.4	10.9	25.0	Refused exercise	1
Hellerstein [9] (1968)	2.0	–	4.5	–	Reports in literature	2.7
Heller [7] (1972)	0.3	1.1	0.4	5.6	Refused exercise, drop-outs	5.0
Rechnitzer [11] (1971)	0.8	1.0	2.4	7.3	Hospital records of Toronto post-MI's	5.0
Bruce [12] (1974)	3.1	10.3	11.2	–	Community experience	4.0
Kavanagh [13, 14] (1980)	2.2	2.1	12.0	10.0	Post-MI non-exercisers	3.0

The nature of the events used to measure therapeutic effect, as well as the naturally occuring frequency of such events in the control group, also influence sample size. For example, when studying the effect of exercise in post-myocardial infarction patients, one could measure therapeutic efficacy in terms of incidence of either fatal recurrences, fatal and non-fatal recurrences, all deaths due to cardiovascular disease, or total deaths from all causes. From the statistical point of view, the latter may be the most desirable, since it represents a true "hard" end-point, or one where there is little room for argument. On the other hand, a clinician is likely to choose deaths from cardiovascular causes as being more appropriate, and, provided the criteria for categorizing such deaths are adequate (autopsy, death certificate, hospital notes, etc.), this is generally acceptable. Myocardial infarction (MI) recurrences, while apparently more pertinent to the question under review, require equally careful identification, and, furthermore, occur less frequently than cardiovascular system (CVS) or total deaths and so increase sample size accordingly. Whichever of these end-points are chosen, the investigator has to be able to predict accurately their naturally occuring incidence in the control group. For instance, if one can anticipate with reasonable assurance that the death rate from cardiovascular causes in the controls will be 5% per annum, then one can select a sample size and follow-up time to allow for such. If we then observe an annual mortality of less than 2% per annum in the treated group (a greater than 50% reduction), we can assume that exercise has been beneficial, and this assumption would have a 95% likelihood of being correct. On the other hand, what if the end of the trial saw only a 1% annual mortality in the control group? The sample size would then be too small to include enough events for a valid conclusion to be drawn. Thus, the accuracy with which an end-point can be measured, as well as the frequency of its occurence, are major components in determining the number of subjects involved in the study.

Drop-out Rate

When all of the above points have been taken into account, there still remains the stumbling block of all prospective studies involving exercise as a therapeutic tool. I refer to the drop-out rate. Strictly speaking, the rules of the randomized trial do not require that a subject *comply* with the mandates of the group to which he is allocated. It is sufficient for statistical purposes merely that he be assigned to that group. Thus, a subject included in the exercise group is counted as an exerciser — whether he exercises or not! (Whether or not he gets fit is considered by the true statistician to be even less relevant). Similarly, a control subject is called a non-exerciser, irrespective of the fact that he has become a fanatical exponent of fitness during the course of the study. To those of us who live in the reality of the clinical world, with all its tangibles and variables, such an approach seems incomprehensible. Nevertheless, if we are to understand the strengths and weaknesses of the randomized trial we must at least be aware of its requirements for validity.

Drop-outs, however, (as opposed to non-compliers) are a different matter. These are individuals who fail to attend a minimum number of classes, e.g. 50% or 60% of those available. Such subjects cannot be counted in the results, and therefore reduce the sample size accordingly. Once again, a realistic prediction of the number of drop-outs must be made in advance of the study, and the corresponding increase made in the sample size. This has invariably been the major weakness of all post-MI exercise rehabilitation trials to date. In the case of the Ontario Multi-Centre trial it was estimated the drop-out rate would not exceed 35%. In actual fact it amounted to 50%.

Recent exercise trials, both non-randomized and randomized, have had to contend with a further major source of programme withdrawal. I refer, of course, to the increasing use of coronary artery bypass graft surgery. Needless to say, intervention of this nature may profoundly affect the outcome in terms of prognosis, and so the recipient must be removed from the study, and is usually labelled a "drop-out".

Other Factors

The major limiting factor in this equation is, of course, money. Budgetary constraints inevitably lead to overly optimistic predictions regarding drop-out rate, with a tendency to "skimp" on the sample size. It has been estimated that the cost of a post-coronary exercise study containing a truly adequate sample size would be in the region of thirty million dollars – a figure unlikely to be provided by any government or private foundation in this age of cutbacks and inflationary trends. In the case of the Ontario Multi-Centre Trial, an extension of the follow-up time to 6, or even 8 years, might well have provided some valid figures. With regard to the National Exercise and Heart Disease Program of the United States (probably the most sophisticated design of any published study to date) budgetary cuts imposed at the onset reduced both sample size and study duration.

Large size studies, of course, have their own peculiar drawbacks. In order to ensure adequate recruitment of subjects a number of centres have to be involved. Often widely spread geographically, there is a tendency for the methods and source of referrals in these centres to vary. Thus, difficulty can be encountered in maintaining standardization of equipment and testing protocol, procedures for exercise and control classes, prevention of contamination between groups (especially difficult in small town centres), etc. Less tangible factors, such as attitude and experience of staff, frequency of staff changeover, and socio-economic backgrounds of subjects, often vary considerably from centre to centre, may be essential elements in overall results, and are well-nigh impossible to control.

What if the randomized trial fails to prove the hypothesis it sets out to test? Can one, then, assume that the hypothesis is incorrect? Only if all of the above conditions have been satisfied. If they have not, then the question remains unanswered. The failure to date of a number of major randomized trials to demonstrate any benefit from exercise can all be explained, as will be seen shortly, on the basis of inadequate sample size, excessive drop-out rates and/or unexpected low recurrence rates in the so-called "control" groups. By the rules of the randomized study, therefore, one cannot say that which has not been proven is untrue.

In point of fact, recent years have seen the whole topic of the clinical trial come under very careful scrutiny. In some cases the conclusions drawn from previously published studies have been challenged as being non-valid, largely because they have ignored some of the ground rules outlined above [15, 16, 17]. However, knowledge can still be gained from the "spoiled" randomized trial. It may be extremely informative to assess the training effect of a particular activity on a group of post-MI patients; or to attempt to define the different outcomes in those who adhere to a programme as opposed to those who do not. Indeed, these observations may be the most valuable clinical contributions the trial has to offer. Strictly speaking, however, such inferences have converted the study from a "randomized" trial to an "observational" study.

Comments on Results of Randomized Multi-Centre Trials

The major randomized trials carried out to date have failed to show the beneficial effects of exercise on post-MI mortality or morbidity (Table 2). In the case of the National Exercise and Heart Disease Project (United States) only the fatal MI recurrence rate approached a statistically significant (P = 0.04) benefit in favour of exercise, and there the principal investigators warned that the choice of such a sub-group for separate consideration must be viewed with considerable reservation.

Interestingly, both the NEHDP and the Ontario Multi-Centre Trial (Canada), show a comparatively low annual mortality in exercise and control groups (less then 2%). In the case of the OMCT, the design assumed incorrectly that there would be a recurrence rate in the controls of at least 5% per annum. Were that to have occurred, there would have been a 90% chance of showing a 50% reduction in the exercise group recurrences, with a probability of 0.05.

The low mortality rates seen in both these studies could possibly be explained as follows:

1. There was unintentional preselection of subjects with a favourable prognosis. The NEHDP protocol included a 6-week preprogramme trial to eliminate those subjects who were likely to be poor adherents; this could conceivably have eliminated the high-risk types.
2. Both control and treatment groups benefited equally from the intervention. In the case of the NEHDP, some 31% of the control group were exercising regularly on their own or at a facility [17]. As for the OMCT, this study was designed to distinguish between the benefits of light as opposed to vigorous exercise, and ideally a third completely sedentary group might have been followed. As it was, the "controls" were all on a walking programme, and in a significant single cohort (100 subjects attending the Toronto Rehabilitation Centres) some 20% were involved in activities such as cross-country skiing, calisthenics, tennis, etc., on a regular basis. Data on the training effect achieved in both programmes showed that in the case of the NEHDP there was little difference between the two groups at the end of the 4-year period, and, in the case of the OMCT, a number of the controls became fitter [22].
3. The post-MI populations' long-term outlook for survival has improved as a result of more beneficial treatment methods and/or lifestyle changes. Unfortunately, evidence to date does not support this conclusion [23].

In all studies the drop-out rates have been in excess of that allowed for by the sample size, and so in all cases the results are as likely due to coincidence or chance as they are to the effects of treatment (Table 3). In the case of the OMCT the sample size was decided on the assumption that the drop-out rate would not exceed 35%. In point of fact it amounted to 50%. The contribution made by surgical intervention (CABG) to this drop-out rate has not been as yet defined.

Table 2. Results of randomized controlled trials

	Exercisers CVS mortality (fatal MI) %	Non-fatal MI %	Controls CVS mortality (fatal MI) %	Non-fatal MI %	N	Duration (years)	P
Kentala (Finland) [18]	14.3 (7.8)	10.2	13.5 (5.0)	12.0	158	2.0	NS
Wilhelmson (Sweden) [19]	18.0 (15.0)	16.0	22.0 (21.0)	18.0	313	4.0	NS
National Exercise and Heart Disease Programme (U.S.A.) [20]	4.6 (0.3)	7.7	7.3 (2.4)	7.6	631	4.0	NS (0.04)
Ontario Multi-Centre Trial (Canada) [21]	(2.1)	7.4	(1.7)	5.6	733	4.0	NS

Table 3. Drop-out rate in randomized controlled trials

	Drop-out rate %	Criteria for "drop-out"
Kentala	85	< 70% attendance
Wilhelmson	70	–
National Exercise and Heart Disease Programme	40 (31% "drop-ins")	< 50% attendance
Ontario Multi-Centre Trial	49	< 60% attendance (or eight consecutive absences from class)

Observational Comments

In the absence of valid conclusions regarding mortality and morbidity, we might make some observations on the above studies. For example, it is of interest that the presence of a consistent and convincing training effect in the various exercising groups is not easy to demonstrate (Table 4). In Kentala's study both active and sedentary improved to the same extent [13]. The Swedish exercisers showed a decrease in heart-rate response to submaximal exercise in only one out of four comparative workloads on the bicycle ergometre, and with data shown for only half of the control group. There was virtually no improvement in aerobic power among the NEHDP exercisers, and while a highly significant reduction of 8.4% in submaximal working heart-rate was recorded, it applied only to some 14% of the exercise group. A further breakdown of both Ontario groups shows a 15% improvement in fitness in those exercisers who were least fit to start with, but only a 5% increase in fitness in those initially most fit. The implication is that the level of physical activity prescribed may have been too low to achieve a consistent training effect. On the other hand, the activities carried out by the "control" group managed to confer a 3.6% increase in fitness on unfit entrants [22]:

In view of the above, one is entitled to ask whether the level of prescribed physical activity in any of the randomized trials to date is too light to train the exercisers, while being at the same time (at least in the case of the Ontario study) sufficiently intense to "contaminate" the sedentary controls. An intriguing alternative possibility, again based on a breakdown of the Ontario figures, is that all we have succeeded in demonstrating so far is the well-known statistical tendency of the data to revert to the mean! In which case, it would probably be more accurate, clinically and statistically, to consider our post-coronary trials to date as being concerned not so much with the effect of *exercise* as with the effect of non-specific *intervention*.

A breakdown of the Ontario groups into trained exercisers and untrained controls reveals a reinfarction rate of 8 in the former and 13 in the latter (Table 5). Taking all trained subjects from both exercise and control groups, and comparing them with all the untrained subjects, we have 10 recurrent MI's in the trained group as opposed to 16 in the untrained (Table 6). There is a trend towards a decrease in recurrence rate in the trained and an increase in the untrained over the period of the study. This is suggestive of the protective effect of training, but obviously the study period would have to be prolonged in order to corroborate this.

Conclusion

In conclusion, the following points should be borne in mind.

1. Successful randomized control trials into the effect of exercise on post-MI patients require large numbers of subjects, involve many centres and need substantial financial support. To completely satisfy all these criteria seems unlikely in view of the current poor state of the economy.
2. Current public world-wide interest in sports and exercise participation militates against the maintenance of a non-exercizing control group for the necessary prolonged time period. The two most recent studies provide excellent examples of the tendency for the controls to indulge in surreptitious regular exercise.

Table 4. Training effect in randomized controlled trials

	Fitness criteria	% Improvement in fitness level		P	Duration (years)
		Exercisers	Controls		
Kentala	Physical work capacity	+ 20	+ 20	NS	2
Wilhelmson	Heart rate, at sub-maximal work-load	+ 6.7	+ 2.6	0.001 (three of four work-loads NS)	4
National Exercise and Heart Disease Programme	Physical work capacity	Virtually 0	0	NS	3
Ontario Multi-Centre Trial	Heart rate, at 1.25 litres/min VO_2	+ 8.4	+ 3.4	.0001	3

Table 5. Reinfarction rates: Trained subjects (exercisers and controls) versus untrained subjects (exercisers and controls) (Ontario Multi-Centre Trial)

Follow-up (years)	Trained subjects reinfarction rate (% per annum)	Untrained subjects reinfarction rate (% per annum)
1	4	4
2	3	5
3	1	4
Total	8	13

Table 6. Reinfarction rates: Trained exercisers versus untrained controls: (Ontario Multi-Centre Trial)

Follow-up (years)	Trained subjects reinfarctions (% per annum)	Untrained subjects reinfarctions (% per annum)
1	7	2
2	3	8
3	0	6
Total	10	16

3. Preselection and non-adherence are factors virtually impossible to control in a free society. Inevitably only a relatively small proportion of available post-MI patients can be prevailed upon to join and remain in the study.
4. Studies involving lifestyle changes contain "soft" variables which are difficult both to identify and to measure objectively. Unlike drug therapy experiments, decisions regarding compliance and treatment effectiveness contain an element of judgment.

In the absence of the unspoiled randomized trail, therefore, we can only advocate the therapeutic use of exercise in post-MI patients for the now universally accepted reason that it brings about marked psychological and physiological improvement. With widespread increase in the use of exercise therapy one can only assume that the accumulated weight of clinical evidence will provide an answer to the question of its effect on prognosis.

References

1   Kavanagh T, Shephard RJ, Tuck JA (1975) Depression after myocardial infarction. Can Med Assoc J 113:23−27
2   Kavanagh T, Shephard RJ, Tuck JA, Qureshi S (1978) Depression following myocardial infarction. The effects of distance running. Ann NY Acad Sci 301:1029−1038
3   Froelicher V (1973) The hemodynamic effects of physical conditioning in healthy young and middle-aged individuals, and in coronary heart disease patients. In: Naughton J, Hellerstein H (eds.) Exercise testing and exercise training in coronary heart disease. Academic Press, New York, p 63
4   Paterson DH, Shephard RJ, Cunningham D, Jones NL, Andrew G (1979) Effects of physical training on cardiovascular function following myocardial infarction. J Appl Physiol 47, 3:482−489
5   Joint Recommendations by the International Society and Federation of Cardiology Scientific councils on Arteriosclerosis, Epidemiology and Prevention, and Rehabilitation (1981) Secondary prevention in survivors of myocardial infarction. BMJ 282
6   Council on Scientific Affairs (1981) Physician-supervised exercise programs in rehabilitation of patients with coronary heart disease. JAMA 245
7   Heller EM (1972) A practical graded exercise program for post-coronary patients − a five year review. Mod Med Can 27:529−542
8   Gottheiner V (1968) Long-range strenous sports training for cardiac reconditioning and rehabilitation. Amer J Cardiol 22:426−435
9   Hellerstein HK (1968) Exercise therapy in coronary disease. Bull NY Acad Med 44:1028−1047
10 Brunner D (1968) Active exercise for coronary patients. Rehab Rec 9:29−31
11 Rechnitzer PA, Pickard HA, Paivio A, Yuhasz MS (1972) Long term follow-up study of survival and recurrence rates following myocardial infarction in exercising and control subjects. Circulation 45:853−857
12 Bruce RA (1974) The benefits of physical training for patients with coronary heart disease. In: Ingelfinger FJ, Ebert RV, Finland M, Relman SWB (eds.) Controvery in Internal Medicine II. Saunders, Philadelphia
13 Kavanagh T, Shephard RJ, Chisholm AW, Qureshi S, Kennedy J (1979) Prognostic indexes for patients with ischemic heart disease enrolled in an exercise-centered rehabilitation program. Amer J Cardiol 44:1230−1240
14 Shephard RJ, Corey P, Kavanagh T (1981) Exercise compliance and the prevention of a recurrence of myocardial infarction. Med & Sci in Sports and Exer 13:1−5
15 Sackett DL, Gent M (1979) Controversy in counting and attributing events in clinical trials. New Engl J Med 301:1410−1412
16 British Medical Journal (1979) The case control study. BMJ 884−885
17 Freiman JA, Chalmers TC, Smith JR, Kuebler RR (1978) The importance of beta, the type II error and sample size in the design and interpretation of the randomized control trial. New Eng Med 299
18 Kentala E (1972) Physical fitness and feasibility of physical rehabilitation after myocardial infarction in men of working age. Ann Clin Res 4 (Suppl 9):1−84
19 Wilhelmsen L, Sanne H, Elmfeldt D, Grimby G, Tibblin G, Wedel H (1975) A controlled trial of physical training after myocardial infarction. Prev Med 4:491−508
20 Naughton J (1980) The effects of physical activity intervention on mortality and morbidity in a post-coronary population. Int Symp on Exer, Fitness and Cardiovascular Health. Oct. 30, 31, Nov. 1, 1980, Tor., Ont., Canada
21 Shephard RJ (1979) Current status and prospects for post coronary exercise multicentre studies. Med & Sci in Sports 11:383−385
22 Shephard RJ (1979) Cardiac rehabilitation in prospect. In: Pollock ML, Schmidt D-H (eds.) Heart disease and rehabilitation. Houghton Miflin, Boston, Mass., p 521−547
23 Weinblatt E, Ruberman W, Goldberg JD, Frank CW, Monk M (1981) Prognosis of men after a first acute myocardial infarction in the 1960's and 1970's: Search for a secular trend. Council on Epidemiology. AHA 30:15

The Reasons for Detrimental Effects of Physical Training on Patients After Myocardial Infarction

R. Rost

Physical training is often considered to be a new method in the treatment of coronary patients. However, the contrary is true. Heberden has already been treating his cardiac patients by exercise. On the other hand, there is no doubt that the introduction of physical training to cardiac patients requires a complete change in the average attitude toward this disease, which carries a lot of psychological problems. Normally these problems are less patient oriented, but rather physician oriented. The patient is used to seeing physical activity as a positive phenomena, however, physicians on the other hand fear that they might endanger their patients by physical stress.

One of the greatest risks of physical exercise, which can be seen at the moment, would be an attitude of uncritical enthusiasm. Keeping the pathologic changes of their patients in mind, it would be wrong — especially from the viewpoint of clinical cardiologists — to conceal the truth, that this movement is not always gratefully welcomed. Such objections must be taken seriously. In the assessment of the value of physical training it is absolutely necessary to balance carefully the benefits against the possible damages. In this paper the reasons for possible detrimental effects should be summarized, including a commentary on the means of avoiding these effects. The following three points form the basis of our discussion:

1. The stimulation of reinfarction or sudden death by physical exercise
2. Stimulation of myocardial insuffiency by chronical overloading
3. Endangering of cardiac patients by a qualitatively or quantitatively incorrecrt training.

Fatal Incidents During Training

The basic presupposition of physical training with cardiac patients is the fact that this treatment will not shorten the patients' lives. However, there are various reports about cardiac arrest during rehabilitation training [1, 2]. In our groups, totaling nearly 200 patients over a time span of 7 years — we witnessed three dramatic events. One case was a fatal reinfarction which occurred during training in the group, another incident was where one patient died suddenly by jogging on his own, and in a third case there was a ventricular fibrillation during long distance skiing, which was successfully treated by defibrillation.

In the face of such events there are a number of questions which have to be asked very carefully. The first question is, are these incidents really caused by physical exercise or are they only statistical events which occur during sports, but are not caused by sports. It should be kept in mind that cardiac patients are dying independently of physical exercise as well. The mortality rate in physically active groups is lower than the normal one in patients after myocardial infarction, considering the fact that they represent selected material. In our groups the mortality rate was 1.5% per year. From the results of the "Hamburg model" it can be concluded that even in a comparison between matched groups of patients, both fufilling the prerequisites for training, the mortality rate of the active group does not exceed the rate of the inactive one [3].

So the statistical answer fails to demonstrate an increased risk of sudden death in physically active groups. On the other hand this answer loses its persuasiveness when it is confronted with the actual incident, even if this is very rare. In such cases not only the physicians, but especially the copatients, and last but not least the lawyer, still question the possible cause of the incident. One of the main advantages of sports, which is generally stressed, is the psychological effect on the patient. Discussing the detrimental effects, however, it should also be stressed that a negative development in a group — the experience of reinfarction or death of colleagues — represents a highly negative effect from the psychological point of view. The most negative experience will be, of course, the actual fatal event during the rehabilitation itself.

These considerations, as well as reports about successfully performed resuscitation during training, lay emphasis on the request that ambulant rehabilitation programms can only be performed under careful medical control. The following conclusions can be drawn: Physical exercise with cardiac patients requires the presence of an experienced physician who is equipped with the necessary emergency devices, including a defibrillator [4]. This condition cannot be temporarily restricted as it is often done [5]. A misunderstanding of coronary heart disease can lead one to consider the cardiac patient to be rehabilitated after, for example, 1 year, and to recommend the patient to participate afterwards in a general sport group. In most cases the anatomic changes are progressing and the risks tend to increase rather than decrease. All our severe incidents occurred in patients who participated for more than 2 years in coronary groups. The consequence of this, which is important, is that patients should take part in medically supervised groups as long as they are willing and able to do so.

Another question, which has to be asked, concerns the possibility of avoiding such incidents by improved preselection procedures. Probably some cases of ventricular fibrillation will be prevented by careful control of exercise arrhythmias through stress testing and tape recording. However, it seems to be unrealistic to request a coronarography, as is sometimes done [6], as a basic examination before participation in physical training.

Risk of Myocardial Overloading

In the case of large myocardial infarction there must be a discussion regarding of physical exercise resulting in an overloading of the remaining myocardium, favoring as a result the development of myocardial insufficiency. This has been shown by case reports in literature. However, the question must be asked: is this detoriation really the consequence of exercise or is it based on the natural progression of the disease?

In our experience we could not observe the development of heart failure in patients participating in the training program. If we consider the enlargement of the heart as a symptom of myocardial insufficiency, this can be demonstrated by the unchanged heart volume of our patients over the years. So we conclude that physical training, on condition that it is performed in a reasonable manner, will not lead to myocardial overloading (Fig. 1).

However, the question should be asked: can heart failure be demonstrated by another method, especially by regularly performed measurements of pulmonary artery pressure? Here we would like to comment on a very frequently discussed problem, that is, should a floating catheter be a presupposition for participation in training or not? This is very often requested, based on the observation that in some cases there is a clear increase in pulmonary artery

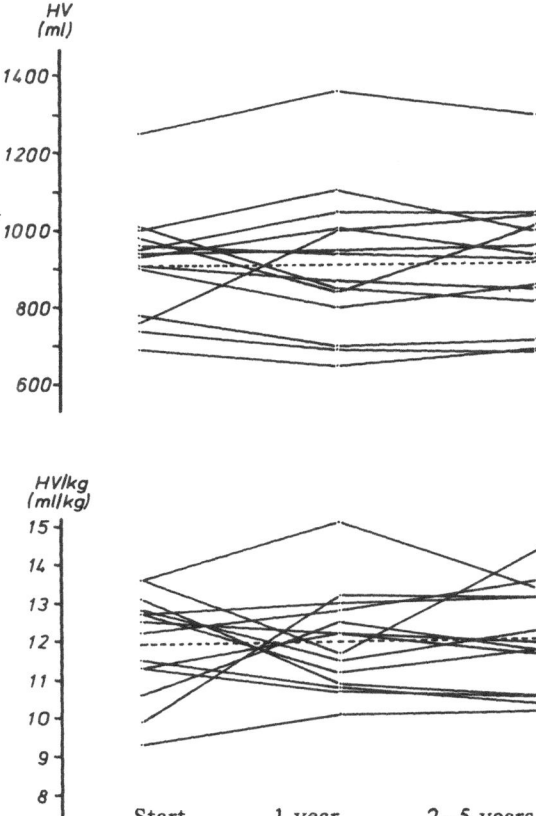

Fig. 1. Observations on cardiac volume in myocardial patients participating in a training program. The upper part demonstrates the absolute volume the lower the HV related to the body weight. The heart volume is not changed after 1 year of training *(center)* or a period of 2–5 years *(right side)* in comparison to its values in the beginning *(left side)*

pressure in spite of a very a high performance capacity and an unchanged stress ECG. On the other hand, the conclusion, which seems to be obvious, namely that these patients could not be trained, cannot yet be substantiated. Up until now we have no data available supporting the suggestion that training will detoriate the prognosis in these cases.

The same is true concerning other parameters, especially ECG. Very often, it is requested, that, for example, patients with large infarction, documented in ECG should not participate in training. But these requests are only based on theoretical considerations. Probably the generally used process of today for the preselection of patients for training will not be sufficient. However, further investigation will be necessary to find out those conditions, which are able to decrease the risk of detoriation as much as possible.

The Risk of Uncritical and Incorrect Training

According to our experience it is not the exercise that endangers the patient, but rather the way in which it is performed, which overburdens the individual both qualitatively or quantitatively. This remark should be elucidated by a number of examples.

In some scientific studies [8, 9] it could be demonstrated that patients after myocardial infarction are even able to run in marathons. This demonstrates that the physical capacity of cardiac patients can be very high, while on the other hand, the question must be asked whether they should really do marathon running? Exercise at such high levels results in a physiologic hyperthrophy of the heart. This means a detoriation of the myocardial oxygen supply, which can be tolerated by a healthy heart within the limits of the critical heart weight, but which can be dangerous for the diseased heart. Conversely, there may exist additional coronary stenosis, which will lead to serious incidents during an exhausting performance. For this reason exercise at high levels by cardiac patients is like playing Russian roulette. Uncritical publications in the nonmedical field suggest to the patient that a more beneficial effect can be obtained from exercise if the load is increased to top levels. These reports are bound to produce fatal incidents (Fig. 2).

One of the main mistakes, which can be observed in cardiac rehabilitation by training, is the uncritical transfer of physiologic knowledge into the pathologic area without regard for its particulars. For this reason training of cardiac patients has to be carefully controlled by cardiologists. Another reason for some of the negative aspects in the development of cardiac rehabilitation is the fact, that, up until now, this development was promoted without sufficient assistance from cardiology. Previously, most clinical cardiologists stood aside and only now have they shown interest in this new field.

In addition to quantitative overloading, many examples of incorrect qualitative exercise can be given. By careful investigation sports medicine has demonstrated useful forms of physical exercise. These principles are often not taken into consideration. There are, for example, ambulant groups, which play such dangerous games as soccer. It is well-known that static

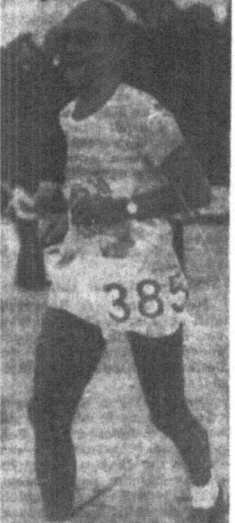

Siegburger Soldat kurierte sich mit Training

Nach dem Herzinfarkt zum Marathonlauf

Auf der langen Strecke wieder gesund geworden

Von unserem Redakteur Norbert Müller

Siegburg (sm) — (53), Siegburger Bürger und Oberstleutnant der Bundeswehr, erlitt im Jahre 1966 einen Herzinfarkt, der ihn zwei Monate ans Bett fesselte. Danach empfahl ihm der Arzt Bewegung und leichte Sportübungen. Seitdem läuft der Offizier Jahr für Jahr etwa 1200

Der gelernte Journalist und Lokalredakteur ging 1963 zur Bundeswehr. Heute betreut er die „Lehr- und Versuchsdienststelle Truppeninformation" der Bundeswehr auf dem Butzweilerhof in Köln. Auch als Offizier arbeitet in seinem gelernten Beruf: Zusammen mit seinen Kameraden stellt er Informationen für Bundeswehr-

Kilometer — beim Training im Siegburger Wald und bei vielen Marathon- und Langstreckenläufen im In- und Ausland. Krönung dieser späten sportlichen Karriere: nahm am „Internationalen Volkslauf Marathon—Athen" teil und schaffte diese klassische Strecke in 4:14:18.

soldaten im Ausland zusammen. Woche für Woche produzieren die Soldaten-Journalisten eine Fernsehaufzeichnung, die über Ampexband an alle bundesdeutschen Truppen im Ausland verschickt wird. Neben Politik und Sport gibt es Informationen aus der Bundeswehr, in dieser Woche natürlich ein Interview des Oberstleutnant

Titel: „Der Marathonlauf".

„Der Herzinfarkt hatte mich gewarnt. Sobald ich einigermaßen fit war, begann ich mit dem Training", berichtete Günter Richter. Der Vater von zwei erwachsenen Söhnen bewohnt ein schmuckes Eigenheim an der

Fortsetzung auf der nächsten Seite

Bundeswehroffizier aus Siegburg, beim Marathonlauf in Griechenland.

Fig. 2. Report in a newspaper recommending marathon running for patients after myocardial infarction

work combined with Valsalva-maneuver may lead to hemodynamic risks. In spite of this fact such exercise is still taken. Another example of questionable exercise uncludes the uncritical recommendation of swimming. Even though this exercise may be useful for cardiac rehabilitation, it can produce severe arrhythmias [10]. Therefore by no means should it be uncritically recommended to all patients.

In summary, it can be pointed out that an optimal training in cardiac rehabilitation requires a careful cooperation of the physician and the physical educator. Thus, extensive information about specific aspects of the partner's field is required. The physical educator must dispose of sufficient medical knowledge and the physician must be informed about the problems of different types of exercise.

Recerences

1   Laubinger G, Bock H (1974) Komplikationen in den Herzinfarkt-Sportgruppen. In: Donat K (ed.) Kardiologische Prävention und Rehabilitation am Wohnort. Perimed, Erlangen

2   Wieser H (1980) Koronarkrankenrehabilitation: Zwischenfälle und Kontroversen bei der Bewegungstherapie. Therapiewoche 30:5218

3   Ilker H (1973) Einrichtung von Herzinfarkt-Sportgruppen am Wohnort. Ärztl Praxis 25:3708

4   Rieger H (1979) Haftungsprobleme in ambulanten Koronarsportgruppen. Dtsch Med Wochenschr 104:1256

5   Halhuber C (1980) Rehabilitation in ambulanten Koronargruppen. Springer, Berlin Heidelberg New York

6   Hellerstein H (1973) Anatomic factors influencing effects of exercise therapy of ASHD subjects. In: Roskamm H, Reindell H (eds.) Das chronisch kranke Herz. Schattauer, Stuttgart New York, p 513

7   Brecht R, Rost R, Behrenbeck D (to be published) Haemodynamische Veränderungen bei Patienten mit KHK ein Jahr nach körperlichem Training. Verh Dtsch Ges Kreislauff

8   Bassler T (1975) Marathon running and immunity to heart disease. The physician and sports medicine 4:77

9   Kavanagh T, Shepard R, Pandti V (1974) Marathon running after myocardial infarction. JAMA 229:1602

10   Samek L, Kirste B, Roskamm H (1977) Herzrhythmusstörungen nach Herzinfarkt. Herz/Kreislauf 9:641

11   Riedel E, Hildebrandt G, Zipp H (1979) Zwischenfälle bei aktiver und passiver Kurbehandlung von Herz-Kreislauf-Kranken. Med Klin 74:199

Does Surgical Therapy Alter the Prognosis of Coronary Heart Disease?

J. von der Emde, R. Hacker, and J. Rein

Coronary surgery is a palliative procedure because coronary heart disease is a metabolic disease leading to a reduction or interruption of myocardial blood flow. The obstructing plaques are frequently in the proximal segments; the distal segments are accessible to the surgeon. The accompanying pain, angina pectoris, does not correlate with the extent of vessel involvement. The intensity is rather dependent on individual sensitivity.

Complete occlusion, usually leading to an infarct, is often caused by thrombosis in a highly stenosed vessel. This usually leads anatomically to myocardial necrosis, eventually in scar tissue, and functionally to rhythm disturbances and eventually to pump failure. The extent of the infarcted myocardial mass depends on the size of the occluded vessel and on the degree of compensation by collaterals and anastomoses. Stenoses of more than 70% cause a perfusion deficit on exercise, which is generally accompanied subjectively by angina pectoris and objectively by signs of ischemia in stress ECG testing (Table 1). If the lumen of coronary artery distal to the proposed anastomoses is over 1.5 mm and the dependent myocardial area still viable with a significant muscle mass involved, the operation, even in single-vessel disease, is promising. Totally occluded vessels with retrograde perfusion and intact perfusion areas leading to significant signs of ischemia in the ECG and severe angina pectoris are an indication for surgery. The above-mentioned prerequisites serve as the basis for an indication to operate, but they must then be modified individually.

The urgency of an operation is determined by five factors, all of which concern the endangered mass of myocardium:

1. Size of the coronary arteries
2. Degree of obstruction
3. Number of vessels narrowed
4. Extent of compensation by collaterals and anastomoses
5. Viability of the endangered muscle mass

Table 1. Indikation for surgery in single-vessel disease

> 70% stenosis
1.5 mm distal lumen diameter
No scar, no akinesis

When the indication for surgery is given the urgency of the procedure increases as the difference between the natural course and operative results becomes greater.

This apparently logical concept must then be proven by statistical studies. On the basis of this statistically verified concept, the individual decision for or against the operation has to be made according to the operative results of a given team, which in turn determine the limits of the operative indication.

To compare the results of medical and surgical therapy, nine parameters should be taken into consideration:

1. Mortality after diagnosis   1 − 5 − 10 years
2. Rate of reinfarction after diagnosis   1 − 5 − 10 years
3. Functional class (NYHA) after diagnosis 1 − 5 − 10 years
4. Physical performance   1 − 5 − 10 years
5. Employability   1 − 5 − 10 years
6. Patency rate of bypass   1 − 5 − 10 years

The results of coronary bypass surgery depend primarily on exact surgical technique. A clearly discernable coronary angiography and left heart ventriculography are absolute prerequisites.

At the Erlangen hospital more than 2800 patients with coronary heart disease have been surgically treated, over 2600 of these with an aortocoronary bypass. The early mortality last year was 1.2%. The results are presented with respect to mortality, functional class, postoperative infarction, and patency rate over a 5-year follow-up period and compared with preoperative data:

1. Age
2. Preoperative myocardial infarction
3. Functional class (NYHA)
4. Ventricular function
5. Ejection fraction
6. Left ventricular end-diastolic pressure
7. Number of diseased vessels
8. Number of bypasses performed
9. Completeness of revascularization
10. Patency rate
11. Distribution of occluded aortocoronary bypasses

The life expectancy in 1581 consecutive patients with saphenous vein coronary artery bypass surgery operated on between 1975 and 1979 at our institution, is compared, in addition, to the survival of 1093 medically treated patients, as published by Lichtlen (Table 2).

Five-year survival was 92.7% in the surgical group versus 71.4% in the medical group. The number of stenosed vessels had much less influence on survival in the surgical then in the medical group. Five-year survival for the patients with single-vessel disease was 97.1% versus 84.6%; for patients with double-vessel disease it was 93.4% versus 67%; and for patients with triple-vessel disease it was 93.5% versus 67%.

Comparing the various age groups, age did not influence early mortality but late mortality was highest in the older age group. However, more elderly patients were free of symptoms or improved. Perioperative and late reinfarction rate was not influenced by age (Table 3).

Table 2. Five-year survival rate for surgical versus medical therapy with I − II − III vessel disease (%)

	Surg.	Med.
I	97.1	84.6
II	93.4	67.0
III	93.5	52.1

As could be expected, patients without preoperative myocardial infarction had a significantly lower late mortality, 8.9% versus 4.9%. The early mortality was not influenced. The same is true for functional improvement (Table 4). Nor was postoperative infarction influenced. The preoperative functional class had an influence on late mortality, 2.8% NYHA II, compared to 14% NYHA IV. Improvement was dependent on preoperative functional class, in that NYHA IV showed only 54.7% symptom-free patients, group I 93.8%. It was similar for the improved cohort. Neither perioperative nor late infarction rate was influenced by functional class.

If revascularization was complete early mortality was not affected; incomplete revascularization markedly influenced late mortality, 3.1% versus 11.2% (Table 5). Surprisingly, there was no influence on the functional class, but a marked influence on late infarction rate, 3.3% versus 9.3%. Most important is patency rate. If all bypasses were patent, early mortality was 2.7% and late mortality was 5.4%. If the bypass was occluded it was 7.0% versus 21.1%. Of the patent group 68.5% were in functional class I (NYHA) and of the occluded group, 43.8%.

The infarction rate was 22.1% in the occluded and 4.7% in the patent group.

Ejection fraction had little influence on the parameters detected. The same holds true for the left ventricular end-diastolic pressure.

Left ventricular function plays a very important role. With a normally functioning ventricle late mortality was 4.1% and with a dyskinetic ventricle, 15.2%. There was no significant influence on functional class, nor on postoperative infarction.

The number of diseased vessels did influence postoperative results. In single-vessel disease, late mortality was 2.9%, in triple-vessel disease 6.5% (Table 6).

Functional class was not affected. This also holds true for postoperative infarction. The number of bypasses performed per patient was without influence on early or late mortality, functional class, or postoperative myocardial infarction.

Table 3. Mortality, functional class, and postoperative myocardial infarction in various age groups

		Mortality Early (30 d) %	Late (5 y) %	NYHA I %	Improved %	Infarction Periop. (30 d) %	Late (5 y) %
Pat.	1 581	1.2	7.3	65.1	87.7	1.0	6.4
Age < 30 years	(5)	0	0	66.7	66.7	0	0
31–40	(102)	0	2.4	66	85	0	7.3
41–50	(490)	0.4	3.4	61.5	83.5	0.6	4.9
51–60	(813)	1.8	6.0	65.2	89.8	1.4	5.2
61–70	(169)	1.2	8.1	76.1	91.8	0.6	2.0
> 70	(2)	0	–	0	100	0	–

Table 4. Mortality, functional class, postoperative myocardial infarction compared to preoperative myocardial infarction and functional class

		Mortality Early (30 d) %	Late (5 y) %	NYHA I %	Improved %	Infarction Periop. (30 d) %	Late (5 y) %
All patients (1 581)		1.2	7.3	65.1	87.7	1.0	6.4
Preop. MI	+ (875)	1.3	8.9	63.4	85.8	1.1	7.1
	0 (687)	1.0	4.9	67.2	90.0	0.6	5.7
NYHA	I (16)	0	0	93.8	–	0	–
	II (205)	0.5	2.8	78.1	78.1	0	3.3
	III (935)	1.0	5.0	66.2	87.7	0.9	7.2
	IV (425)	2.1	14.0	54.7	93.4	1.4	6.6

Table 5. Mortality, functional class, postoperative myocardial infarction compared to completeness of revascularization and bypass patency

	Mortality		NYHA		Infarction	
	Early (30 d)	Late (5 y)	I	Improved	Periop. (30 d)	Late (5 y)
	%	%	%	%	%	%
All patients (1 581)	1.2	7.3	65.1	87.7	1.0	6.4
Revascularization						
complete (892)	1.0	3.1	66.6	88.3	0.6	3.3
incomplete (689)	1.5	11.2	63.2	86.8	1.5	9.3
Patency rate						
bypass patent + (377)	2.7	5.4	68.5	88.0	1.3	4.7
bypass occluded (57)	7.0	21.1	43.8	75.0	5.4	22.1
0						

Table 6. Mortality, functional class, postoperative myocardial infarction compared to diseased vessels and number of bypasses performed

	Mortality Early (30 d)	Mortality Late (5 y)	NYHA I	Improved	Infarction Periop. (30 d)	Infarction Late (5 y)
	%	%	%	%	%	%
All patients (1 581)	1.2	7.3	65.1	87.7	1.0	6.4
No. of vessels diseased						
1 (325)	0.9	2.9	65.3	83.3	0.6	4.5
2 (480)	1.0	4.9	64.1	87.3	0.6	5.2
3 (598)	1.0	6.5	63.4	88.2	1.3	5.6
left main (178)	2.8	9.5	73.9	95.7	1.1	4.2
No. of ACB performed						
1 (564)	1.1	5.4	62.6	83.2	0.7	5.9
2 (715)	1.7	6.9	64.4	89.0	1.4	5.1
3 (280)	0.4	1.6	70.7	92.4	0.4	1.9
4 (19)	0	—	84.2	94.7	0	0
5 (3)	0	—	66.7	100.0	0	—

Do Recent Changes in Medical Therapy Alter the Prognosis in Coronary Heart Disease?

K. Bachmann

Are recent changes in medical therapy capable of improving long-term survival in coronary heart disease? This is a basic question in the controvery between medical and surgical treatment of a disease which is still number one in life table analysis. At the present state of operative treatment of coronary heart disease the majority of centers perform the venous bypass [14] and the internal mammary anastomosis (Green 1972) with an operative mortality below 2%, and less than 5% perioperative myocardial infarction and a more than 90% patency rate of the transplants [9, 22, 16. 25, 27, 23, 15, 21].

This progress in the operative treatment of coronary heart disease has brought the cumulative 5-year survival rate to 90% and above. These advances in the operative treatment of coronary heart disease are not limited to good-risk patients but also include patients with three vessel disease and moderate impairment of the left ventricular pump function. In the early stage of direct myocardial revascularization these patients had a high mortality rate and the same poor long-term prognosis as under medical treatment. Today it is our policy to reject patients with an ejection fraction of less than 30% from bypass surgery, because in this situation no myocardium is left to be revascularized. Operative treatment in this situation adds only a risk without offering the chance of postoperative improvement of symptoms and cardiac performance.

Direct myocardial revascularization was criticized from the very beginning as far as long-term survival is concerned. Today those who compare bypass surgery with "a pill which at that time no one would prescribe" [7] or criticized it to be experimental and at the crossroads [4] are opposed to the criticism of their colleges, who declare that the venous transplant and the internal mammary implant may improve not only quality of life but also life expectancy [23, 9, 16, 22, 21, 25]. However, we must bear in mind that medical therapy has also changed during the last decade of bypass surgery. It is debatable whether this had the effect of improving the survival rate as compared to the studies of Bruschke 1973 [6] and Burgraf and Parker 1975 [8], which served as reference for evaluating operative treatment.

The negative attitude toward operative treatment may be explained on the basis of the high mortality rate and perioperative myocardial infarction rate demonstrated in the early 70s by Bertolasi 1974 [3], Conti 1975 [10], Selden 1975 [32], Mathur 1975 [27], Kloster 1975 [26], and Murphy 1977 [28]. At the same time medical therapy changed rapidly, introducing beta-adrenergic blockers, nitrate esters, calcium antagonists, and platelet active drugs. Thus medical therapy has become more effective in improving the symptomatic status and working capacity of patients with coronary heart disease. Nevertheless the question still remains to be answered: have these advances in medical treatment resulted in prolonging life and is coronary surgery still at the crossroad (Braunwald 1977) [4]?

This question needs a stratified discussion under different aspects:

First. A great number of trials concluded and under way studying the randomized long-term effect of platelet active drugs, coumarine, and beta blockers have to be discussed.

Second. Treatment of a coronary patient in daily practice is quite different from treatment in prospective randomized trials. The patient in such a long-term study will benefit from continuous supervision so that even the placebo group will have a better prognosis. Furthermore dosis in general practice have a greater variation and the patients compliance is less as compared to clinical studies. Therefore it is basically questionable whether benefits in a trial even on a statistical significant level will be the same in general practice.

Third. Through the years the ideas of rehabilitation and social medicine for primary and secondary prevention of coronary heart disease have grown, and the effect of rehabilitation on long-term survival has to be taken into consideration in interpreting chances in survival in patients who are under medical treatment.

Long-term Trials. If we look at the beta blockers, one of the most experienced experts in this field came to the pessimistic conclusion in 1979 that around 30 million dollars are now spent annually with little benefit to science and patients [33]. Randomized multicenter trials demonstrate a trend toward lower mortality, but these findings have not been statistically significant [2, 5, 8, 12, 14, 17, 19, 29, 32, 34]. Beside this there exists no general accepted recommendation regarding the ideal candidate, the optimal dose, and the beginning and the end of beta-blocking therapy. The question of what drug should be administered at what stage of coronary heart disease and what are the criteria for terminating beta blockade are still open.

The same situation exists when we look at the trials which deal with the platelet inhibitors [1, 2, 5, 11, 12, 13, 29].

The question whether or not the patient with coronary heart disease will benefit from aspirin or sulfinpyrazone still remains open. Again, in the eight studies with platelet active drugs there is a trend toward prolongation of life by primary or secondary prevention of "ischemic events", but the results are not statistically significant. But overlooking all statistics the concept of platelet active drugs is still not conclusive as to its consequence for long-lasting treatment. Even positive results such as in the Germany-Austrian Aspirin trial [5, 8] have to be criticized when looking at the opposite results in the different participating hospitals. Furthermore one should emphasize that a subgroup of the Heidelberg trial treated with phenbrocoumon had a higher total mortality as compared to the placebo group. The anturano trial demonstrated reduction of a total mortality over 16 months of 32% which was borderline statistically significant but restricted to the prevention of sudden death during the first 6 months [4]. This Anturano Reinfarction Trial indicates the problem of starting and terminating primary and secondary prevention by drugs. Thus at the present state of medical treatment the evaluation of beta blockers, calcium antagonists, and platelet active drugs in terms of prevention of ischemic events and cardiac death is not conclusive, and routine use is still speculative and experimental. No general accepted evidence exists that medical therapy has improved long-term prognosis to a degree comparable to the annual attrition rate reported from postoperative follow-up after direct myocardial revascularization procedures.

Long-term Follow-up Under Medical Treatment. The findings of the literature and our own experience in the long-term prognosis of coronary heart disease confirm this statement. There are essentially two proofs that make it unlikely that medical treatment has improved long-term prognosis during the last 2 decades. A 10-year follow-up of coronary patients classified at the Cleveland Clinic angiographically, between 1963 and 1965, has shown no leveling off in the survival curve of this population at the point when medical therapy changed significantly [30] (Fig. 1). Second, the annual attrition rate remained at 4% regardless of the changes in medical therapy in comparison with studies by ourselves and others over the last 50 years [18, 24, 31].

Our own material consists of 984 patients who were treated medically and followed-up between 1969 and 1977. The total cummulative 5-year survival rate was 68.2% and thus in the range for groups treated in the 70's. The survival curve of our own group is almost the same as that reported by Proudfit [30] for patients treated 10 years earlier before beta blockers, platelet active drugs, long-acting nitrates, and calcium antagonists became availble in general practice. The survival rate in our study varies according to the severity, extent, and location of coronary lesions and whether impairment in left ventricular pump function, documented by the ejected fraction, is present or not. In the functional class 2 of our grading system, which includes patients with one or two vessel disease but a normal left ventricular function, the 5-year survival rate is 89.2% (Fig. 2). It decreased to 11.4% in patients with three or four vessel disease and a critically reduced left ventricular pump function indicated by an ejection of 30% or below. So our survival curves lead to the same conclusion as the Cleveland long-term trial in that medical therapy has not altered the long-term prognosis. This is in agreement with three American studies separated by almost half a century demonstrating an annual mortality rate of approximately 4% [18, 24, 31]. We must not forget that problems of prescription and patient compliance in general practice may account for this lack

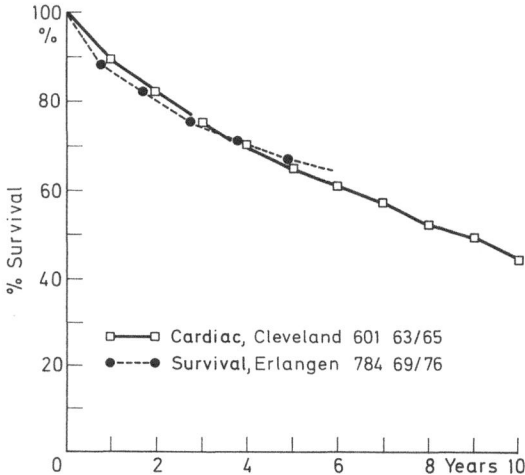

Fig. 1. Survival curves of 601 male patients with coronary heart disease reported by the Cleveland Clinic superimposed on the survival curve of our own long-term follow-up of 784 men. The medical treatment of the Cleveland group started between 1963 and 1965 after the diagnosis had been established angiographically and between 1969 and 1975 in the Erlangen group.Thus the cumulative survival rate in the first 5 years of observation represents the prognosis of patients before and after basic changes in medical treatment by introduction of beta blockers, platelet active drugs, long-acting nitrates, and calcium antagonists had taken place. Both curves are close to each other and demonstrate that changes in medical treatment have not changed life expectancy of patients who are treated in general practice

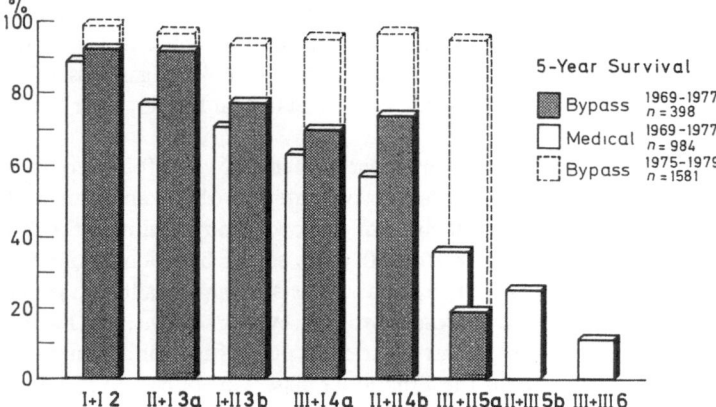

Fig. 2. Five-year cumulative survival rate of patients during medical treatment and after aortocoronary bypass surgery. The survival rate of patients treated medically has not changed as compared to trials during the last 50 years. In the late 70s myocardial revascularization has improved life expectancy, offering a 5-year survival rate of more than 90% regardless of the preoperative severity of coronary artery disease and impairment of left ventricular function. The grading system considers the severity of coronary artery lesions and impairment in left ventricular function (class 2 = 1–2 vessel disease and normal left ventricular ejection fraction; class 6 = 4 vessel disease and left ventricular ejection fraction of 30% or less)

of improvement. To elucidate this problem we have analyzed the medical treatment of patients with angiographically diagnosed coronary heart disease in the years 1970, 1975, and 1980 (Fig. 3). It turned out that in both groups, patients with coronary heart insufficiency only and patients after myocardial infarction, the use of short- and long-acting nitrates has increased while coronary vasodilators, which were the dominating drugs in 1970, are no longer important, in daily practice. Beta blockers are accepted more and more as a basic drug in the treatment of symptoms and arrhythmias as well as in the still speculative primary and secondary prevention of myocardial infarction. Furthermore, it turns out that digitalis is administered more critically.

Summary

Todays standard medical treatment has improved the management of the symptoms, but we are still a long way from claiming that we have a pill which prolongs the life expectancy of the patient with coronary heart disease. This lack is partly due to the drugs presently available and partly due to the special situation in everyday practice, which seems to be quite different from prospective randomized multicenter studies. At the present time, in a patient with operable multivessel disease and no critically depressed left ventricular function, the venous transplant and internal mammary anastomoses is the better offer compared to medical treatment. Medical and operative treatment of coronary heart disease may not be seen in competition. Coronary insufficiency at rest, myocardial infarction, and sudden death are the

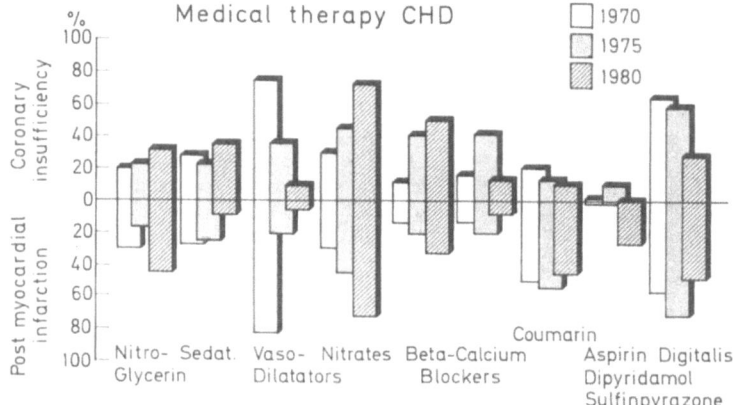

Fig. 3. Changes in the prescription of drugs in general practice between 1970 and 1980. Statistics are based on 100 consecutive patients for each year

endpoints of progressive coronary atherosclerosis. What the patient needs is a more differentiated approach, adding medical treatment and bypass surgery at the right time to the basic measures of prevention and rehabilitation.

References

1 Anturano Reinfarction Trial Research Group (1978) Sulfinpyrazone in the prevention of cardiac death after myocardial infarction. N Engl J Med 298:289
2 Aspirin Myocardial Infarction Study Research Group (1980) The aspirin myocardial infarction study: final results. Circulation 62 (Suppl V)
3 Bertolasi CA, Tronge JE, Carreno CA, Jalon J, Vega MR (1974) Unstable angina: Prospective randomized study of its evolution, with and without surgery. Am J Cardiol 33:201
4 Braunwald E (1977) Coronary-artery surgery at the crossroads. N Engl J Med 297:661
5 Breddin K, Loew D, Lechner K, Überla K, Walter E (1979) Secondary prevention of myocardial infarction. Comparison of acetylsalicylic acid, phenprocoumon and placebo. A multicenter two-year prospective study. Thromb Haemostas 40:225
6 Bruschke AVG, Proufit WL, Sones FM (1973) Progress study of 590 consecutive non-surgical cases of coronary disease followed 5–9 years. I. Arteriographic correlations. Circulation 47:1147
7 Burch GE (1971) Coronary artery surgery-saphenous vein bypass. Am Heart J 82:137
8 Burggraf GW, Parker JO (1975) Prognosis in coronary artery disease: Angiographic, hemodynamic, and clinical factors. Circulation 51:146
9 Cohn LH, Collins JJ (1979) The effect of coronary bypass on longevity – A nonrandomized study. In: Roskamm H, Schmutziger M (eds) Coronary heart surgery. Springer, Berlin Heidelberg New York, p 13
10 Conti CR, Gilbert JB, Hodges M, Hutter AM, Kaplan E, Newell J, Resnekov L, Rosati R, Ross RS, Russel RO, Schroeder JS, Wolk M (1975) Unstable angina pectoris: Randomized study of surgical versus medical therapy: National cooperative unstable angina pectoris study group. Am J Cardiol 35:129
11 Coronary Drug Project Research Group (1980) Aspirin in coronary heart disease. Circulation 62 (Suppl V)

12 Elwood PC, Williams WO (1979) A randomized controlled trial of aspirin in the prevention of early mortality in myocardial infarction. J R Coll Gen Pract 29:413
13 Ellwood PC, Cochrane AL, Burr ML, Sweetnam PM, Williams G, Welsby E, Hughes SJ, Retnon R (1974) A randomized controlled trial of acetylsalicylic acid in the secondary prevention of mortality from myocardial infarction. Brit Med J 1:436
14 Favaloro RG (1968) Saphenous vein autograft replacement of severe segmental coronary artery occlusion — operative technique. Ann Thorac Surg 5:334
15 Favaloro RG (1979) Direct myocardial revascularisation, a ten year journey. Am J Cardiol 43:109
16 Flemma RJ (1979) The effects of aortocoronary bypass surgery on life expectancy — A nonràndomized study. In: Roskamm H, Schmutzinger M (eds) Coronary Heart Surgery. Springer, Berlin Heidelberg New York, p 18
17 Fox KM, Chopra MP, Portal RW, Aber CP (1975) Long-term beta blockade; possible protection from myocardial infarction. Br Med J 1:117
18 Frank CW, Weinblatt E, Shapiro S (1973) Angina pectoris in men. Circulation 47:509
19 Green GE (1972) Internal mammary artery-to-coronary artery anastomosis. Ann Thorac Surg 14:260
20 Green KG (1975) Improvement in prognosis of myocardial infarction by long-term beta-adrenoreceptor blockade using practolol. A multicenter international study. Br Med J 11:735
21 Hacker RW, Torka M, v d Emde J (1981) Lebenserwartung nach aortakoronarem Bypass. Jahrestg Dtsch Ges Thorax-, Gefäßch. Bad Nauheim
22 Haller RJ, Cooley DA, Garcia E, Mathur VS, de Castro CM (1979) Does coronary bypass surgery prolong life expectancy? In: Roskamm H, Schmutziger M (eds) Coronary Heart Surgery. Springer, Berlin Heidelberg New York, p 26
23 Hammermeister KE, de Roven TA, Dodge HT (1979) Evidence from a nonrandomized study that coronary surgery prolongs survival in patients with two-vessel disease. Circulation 59:430
24 Kannel WB, Feinleib M (1972) Natural history of angina pectoris in the Framinham Study. Prognosis and survival. Amer J Cardiol 29:154
25 Karp RB, Kouchoukos NT, Kerklin JW (1979) Factors to prolong survival in patients with coronary heart disease. In: Roskamm H, Schmutzinger M (eds) Coronary Heart Surgery. Springer, Berlin Heidelberg New York, p 36
26 Kloster F, Kremkau L, Rahimtoola S, Griswold H, Ritzmann L, Neill W, Starr A (1975) Prospective randomized study of coronary bypass surgery for chronic stable angina. Circulation 52:90
27 Mathur VS, Hall RJ, Garcia E, de Castro CM, Cooley DA (1980) Prolonged life with coronary bypass in patients with three-vessel disease. Circulation 62 (Suppl I):1–90
28 Murphy ML, Hultgren HN, Detre K, Thomsen J, Takaro T (1970) Treatment of chronic stable angina. A preliminary report of survival data of the Randomized Veterans Administration Cooperative Study. N Engl J Med 297:621
29 Persantin-Aspirin Re-Infarction Study (1980) The persantin-aspirin reinfarction study. Persantin and aspirin in coronary heart disease. Circulation 62:449
30 Proudfit WL, Bruschke AV, Sones FM (1978) Natural history of obstructive coronary artery disease: ten-year study of 601 nonsurgical cases. Prog. Cardiovasc Dis 21:53
31 Richards DW, Bland EF, White PD (1956) A complete twenty-five-year follow-up study of 456 patients with angina pectoris. J Chon Dis 4:423
32 Selden R, Neill WA, Ritzmann LW, Okies JE, Anderson RP (1975) Medical versus surgical therapy for acute coronary insufficiency: A randomized study. N Engl J Med 293: 1329
33 Vedin JA, Wilhelmsson CE (1979) A review of current beta-blocker trials in the world. Hart Bull 10:180
34 Wilhelmsson CE, Vedin JA, Wilhelmsen L, Tibblin G, Werkö L (1974) Reduction of sudden death after myocardial infarction by treatment with alprenolol. Lancet II:1158

Long-Term Effects of Aortocoronary Bypass Surgery of Exercise Tolerance and Vocational Rehabilitation

H. Gohlke, Ch. Gohlke-Bärwolf, K. Schnellbacher, K. Heidecker,
L. Samek, L. Görnandt, P. Stürzenhofecker, and H. Roskamm

There is general agreement that aortocoronary bypass surgery improves angina pectoris in a high percentage of patients (Council on Scientific Affairs 1979). There is also agreement that in certain subgroups of patients survival is improved through the revascularization procedure (Gunnar et al. 1980). There is less agreement as to whether the improved quality of life is reflected in a high return-to-work rate after bypass surgery (Wallwork et al. 1978; Lichtlen et al. 1978; Blümchen et al. 1979; Oberman and Kouchoukos 1979).

This study attempts to answer the following questions:

1. Is the improvement of angina pectoris associated with an objective increase of exercise tolerance?
2. For how long is the improved exercise tolerance maintained after aortocoronary bypass surgery?
3. Does the improved exercise tolerance lead to a higher return-to-work rate?

Patient Material and Methods

Between 1973 and 1978, 902 patients examined pre- and postoperatively in the Rehabilitationszentrum Bad Krozingen, Germany, underwent aortocoronary bypass surgery without associated procedures.

In February 1979 all patients were evaluated by questionaire concerning their current work status.

Sixty-four patients had died; 58 questionnaires were not returned or were incomplete; all these 58 patients were known to be alive.

Of the remaining 780 patients 467 were 55 years or younger at the time of operation. The study population of age 55 or younger at the time of operation was chosen to exclude patients who could retire because of reaching the age limit rather than for medical reasons within the follow-up period. Although some of these patients will reach age 60 during the 5-year follow-up. All patients had undergone pre- and postoperative exercise testing. An average of 2.9 exercise tests per patient were performed between 1 und 5 years after surgery and were available for review. All exercise tests were performed in the supine position with an electrically braked bicycle ergometer until fatique, angina pectoris, 80% of the age-predicted maximal heart rate, or more than 0.4 MV of ST segment depression occurred.

Coronary angiography and left ventriculography was performed using Sones' or Judkins' technique. A more than 50% narrowing of the luminal diameter of one of the three main vessels was considered a significant lesion.

Left ventricular angiography was performed in the 30° right anterior oblique projection, where the left ventricule was divided into five segments (anterobasal, anterolateral, apical, diaphragmal, posterobasal), and in the left anterior oblique projection, where the left ventricle was divided into a septal and a posterolateral segment.

Left ventricular function was graded on a scale of 1 to 4 depending on the number of hypo- or akinetic segments.

Left ventricular function with 1 mildly hypokinetic segment was still considered normal, with 1 or 2 hypo- or akinetic segments as midly impaired. With 3 or more hypo- or akinetic segments left ventricular function was considered moderately impaired, and severe impairment of left ventricular function was considered to be present when nearly all segments showed severe hypo- or akinesis. The degree of revascularization was determined angiographically one year after surgery in 437 patients. Revascularization was considered complete if all lesions of over 50% narrowing in a bypassable vessel were provided with an open graft. It was considered sufficient if at least the main vessel supplying the left ventricle was provided with an open graft, as incomplete if the graft to the main vessel of the left ventricle was occluded but at least one additional graft was open. The revascularisation procedure was considered a total failure when all constructed grafts were occluded.

Results

The preoperative exercise tolerance in these 467 patients was 65 W and increase to 95 W at 1 year after surgery. Exercise tolerance decreased only slowly to 85 W over the next 4 years (Fig. 1).

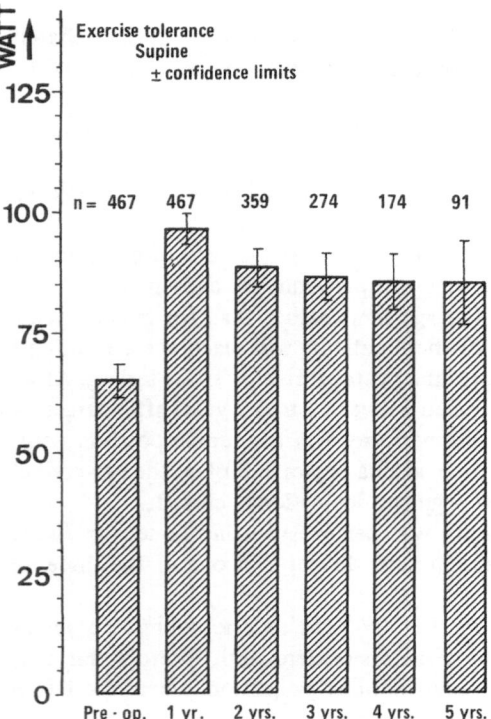

Fig. 1. Exercise tolerance before and 1 to 5 years after bypass surgery (467 patients age 55 or younger)

The amount of exercise that could be performed without the occurrence of angina pectoris more than doubled from 41 W prior to surgery to 86 W 1 year after surgery; there was a slow decline to 68 W of angina-free exercise tolerance at 5 years after surgery.

The work status of these patients from 1 to 5 years after surgery is shown in Fig. 2: approximately 50%–55% of patients were back to work from 1 to 4 years after surgery and slightly less than 50% at 5 years. The percentage of patients retired increases slowly whereas the percentage of patients reports as sick declined slowly from 12% to 5%.

To determine the influence of physical job demands on the return-to-work rate, our patients were divided into two groups: patients engaged in physical labor on their job and patients without physical labor. These groups are referred to as blue-collar and white-collar workers respectively.

Prior to surgery the two groups did not differ significantly with respect to age, exercise tolerance, ST segment depression during exercise, the maximal double product of heart rate and blood pressure achieved during exercise, the percentage of patients with single, double and triple vessel disease, and the degree of left ventricular dysfunction in the pre-operative left ventricular angiogram (Table 1). Also the degree of revascularization achieved was comparable in both groups. In both groups exercise tolerance after surgery was significantly improved compared to preoperative tolerance, and this was maintained in both groups until 5 years after surgery; however, white-collar workers had a significantly better exercise tolerance throughout the entire 5-year follow-up period (Fig. 3).

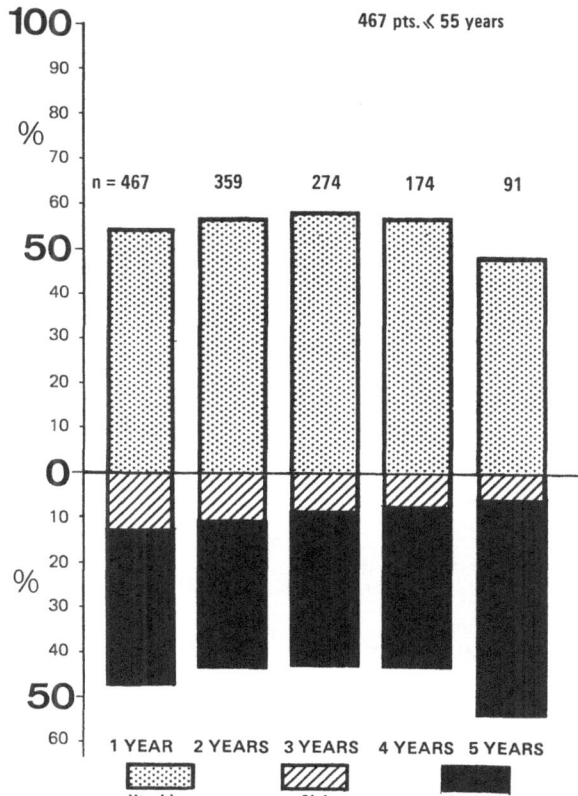

Fig. 2. Working status 1 to 5 years after ACBS

Table 1. Preoperative characteristics in blue- and white-collar workers

Aortocoronary bypass surgery in patients $\leqslant 55$ years	Blue collar n = 230	White collar n = 237
Mean age	47.8 ± 0.6	49.0 ± 0.6
Exercise tolerance in watts	60.0 ± 4.0	65.0 ± 4.0
ST $\downarrow \geqslant 0.1$ mV	n = 201	n = 202
	0.26 ± 0.02	0.26 ± 0.01
HF x RR$_{syst}$ x 10^{-2}	184 ± 7	188 ± 7
1/2/3 VD	10/36/54%	12/30/57%
LV-function norm. or mildly impaired	80%	80%
mod. or severely impaired	20%	20%

The maximal double product during exercise testing tended to be lower in the blue-collar workers throughout the follow-up period, although this difference did not reach statistical significance (Fig. 4). The reason for the less favorable functional results of aortocoronary

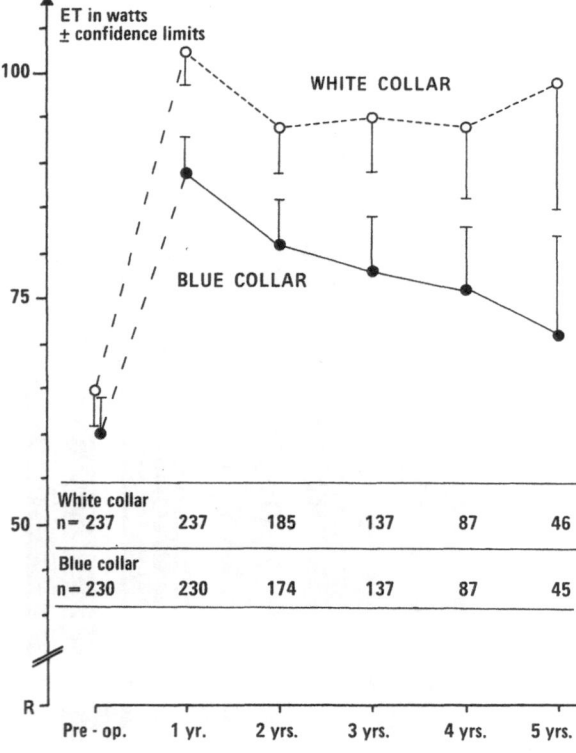

Fig. 3. Exercise tolerance 1 to 5 years after surgery (blue and white collar workers)

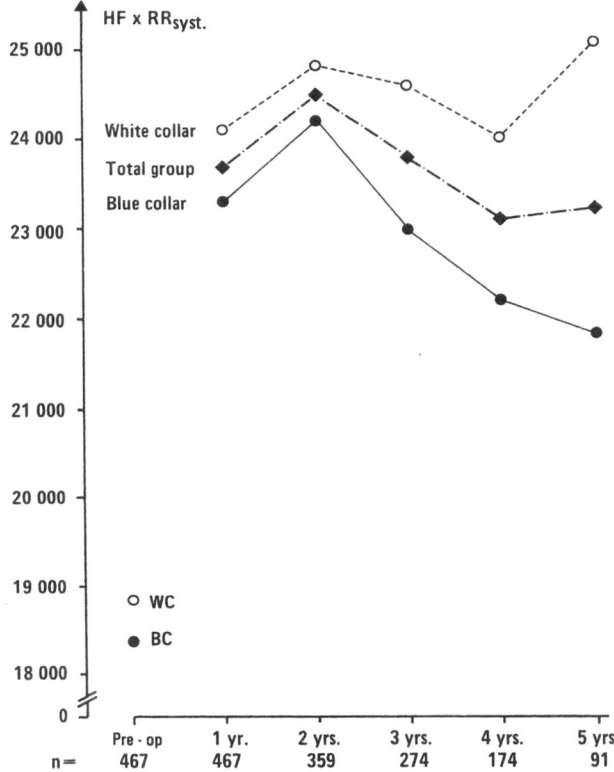

Fig. 4. Maximal double product 1 to 5 years after ACBS

bypass in blue-collar workers is not entirely clear at present, but probably reflects better conditioning in white-collar workers.

The percentange of patients working at 1 through 5 years after surgery is shown in Fig. 5 for blue- and white-collar workers. The percentage of patients working was consistently lower in the blue-collar group; conversely the percentage of patients retired was consistently higher.

A correlation of the postoperative exercise tolerance with the percentage of patients back to work is shown in Fig. 6a and b. Patients are divided into 4 groups according to their post-operative exercise tolerance of less than 60 W, 60–90 W, 90–120 W, or more than 120 W. The lines connect the patient groups at the follow-up intervals indicated. There is a clear-cut relation between exercise tolerance and return-to-work rate throughout the entire follow-up period both for blue-collar workers (Fig. 6a) and for white-collar workers (Fig. 6b).

Analyzing only exercise tolerance regardless of the time intervall after surgery the following relationship can be shown (Fig. 7):

In both blue- and white-collar workers (Table 2) there is a statistically highly significant rela-tionship between exercise tolerance and return-to-work rate ($p < 10^{-7}$).

Below an exercise tolerance of 120 W after surgery, blue-collar workers have a 10%–20% lower return-to-work rate than white collar workers with similar exercise tolerance.

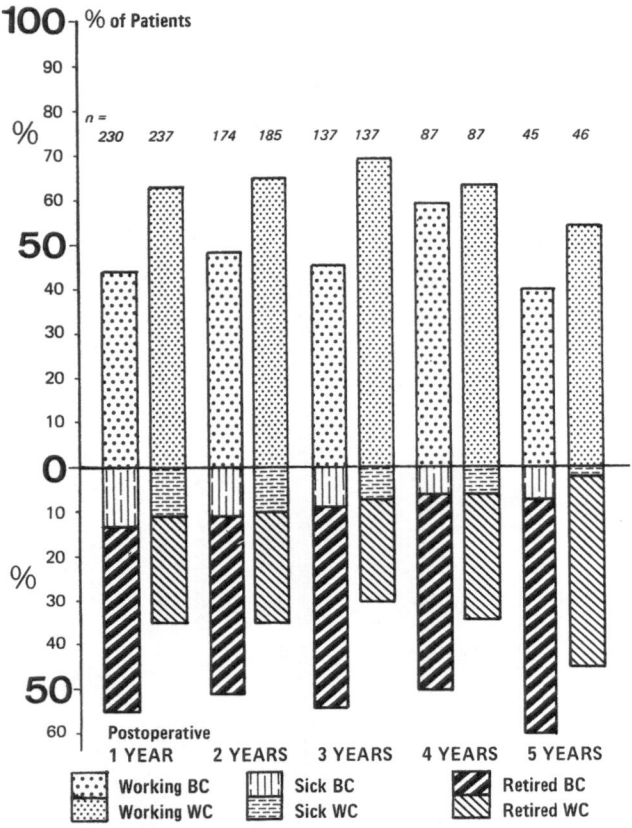

Fig. 5. Working status of blue and white collar workers at 1 through 5 years after bypass surgery (*BC*, blue collar; *WC*, white collar), (n = 467 ≤ 55 years old)

If the exercise tolerance exceeds 120 W, there is no longer a difference in return-to-work rate between blue-collar and white-collar workers. In both groups 75% of patients are back to work after surgery.

Apart from the exercise tolerance we have also looked at other pre- and postoperative parameters, listed in tables 3 and 4; these data have been published previously (Schnellbacher et al. 1980); significant differences between patients working and retired were found with respect to the number of patent grafts and accordingly the degree of revascularization, the absence of postoperative angina pectoris and the degree of left ventricular dysfunction postoperatively as determined angiographically.

Discussion

Other factors than the medical outcome after bypass surgery influence significantly the return-to-work rate: preoperative work status, age, educational level (Rimm et al. 1976; Niles et al. 1980), the attitude of the employer, the motivation of the individual patient, the

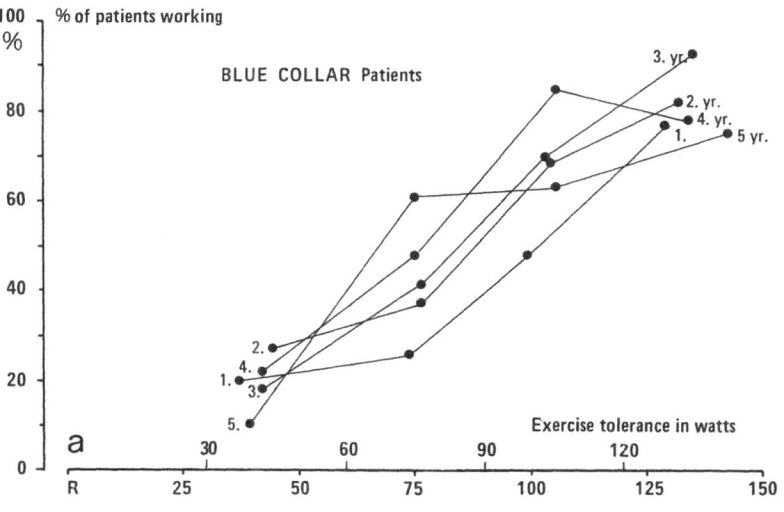

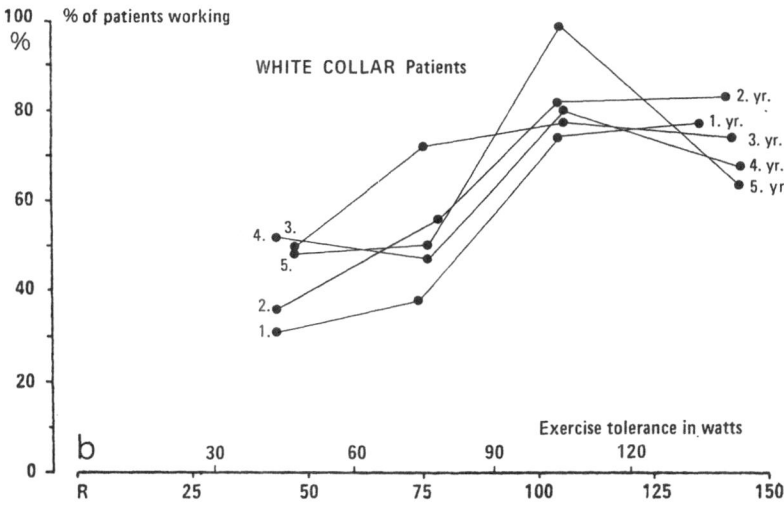

Fig. 6a, b. Patients working 1 to 5 years postop. in relation to ET

retirement benefits, the medical insurance system, and the current unemployement rate are factors to be considered (Barnes et al. 1977; David 1979; Oberman and Kouchoukos 1979; Kass Wenger and Hurst 1980). Therefore it is difficult to compare the return-to-work rate in different countires because the social systems may differ. The reported return-to-work rates in larger series from the United States (Hammermeister et al. 1979; Lawrie et al. 1977) and from Scotland (Wallwork et al. 1978) are significantly higher than in series reported in the German literature and also higher than our own experience. This is probably due to different patient selection and differences in the social system.

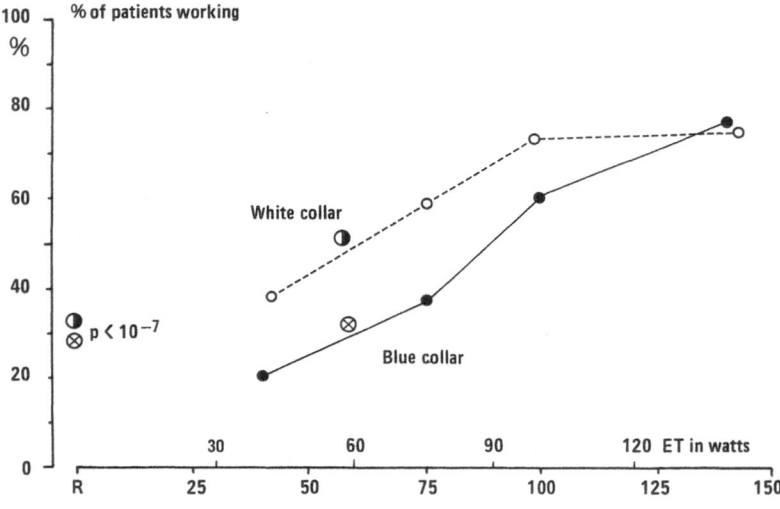

Fig. 7. Patients working in relation to ET (n = 467)

Previous publications on German patient populations could not show a significant influence of the medical outcome after bypass surgery on the return-to-work rate (Blümchen et al. 1979; Lichtlen et al. 1978). The symptomatically improved patients showed only a slightly higher return to work rate than patients with persisting angina (Benesch et al. 1979). It was also suggested that patients going through a rehabilitation program have a lower return-to-work rate than others (Benesch et al. 1979). Our results differ from these reports in the literature and indicate that within the framework of a comprehensive rehabilitation program the medical outcome after aortacoronary bypass surgery has a highly significant influence on the return-to-work rate. Exercise tolerance after bypass surgery was significantly improved for 5 years and correlated well with the return-to-work rate not only 1 year after surgery but throughout the entire follow-up period of 5 years; 75% of patients with an exercise tolerance of more than 120 W will return to work in blue-collar as well as in white-collar groups; these results are still far from satisfactory, but they indicate that the medical outcome has a high priority in determining who returns to work; this can be considered a success or rehabilitation that is oriented toward functional evaluation of the patient. An optimal surgical results with a revascularization that is as complete as possible is a prerequisite for good functional results and successful vocational rehabilitation.

Table 2. Degree of revascularization in blue- and white-collar workers as determined by angiography at 1 year after surgery

	Blue c. n = 218	White c. n = 219
Compl. of sufficient	83%	81%
Incompl. or total failure	17%	19%

Table 3. Preoperative parameters in patients working after surgery and in those retired

	Working n = 225	Retired n = 143	Signific.
Age	50.6 yrs.	53.0 yrs.	
Myoc. inf.	66.2%	73.4%	
max. watts	67.4 w	57.6 w	
max. ST ↓	0.23 mV	0.19 mV	∅
max. PCW	27.3 mmHg	25.8 mmHg	
1/2/3 VD	12.3/31.1/56	6/31.3/61.5%	
LV-funct.	29.3/54.4	28.7/51%	
(0/1/2)	18.2%	20.3%	

Table 4. Postoperative parameters in patients working after surgery and in those retired

	Working n = 225	Retired n = 143	Signific.
Grafts/pt.	2.52	2.49	∅
Open gr./pt.	2.10	1.70	+
Revascularization			
(1 + 2/3 + 4)	85.3/14.6	72.9/27.0%	++
Free of AP	85.8%	54.9%	++
max. watts	102.4 w	79.3 w	++
Post. op. LV-			
function 0	28.4%	20.8%	
1	53.3%	50.7%	++
2	18.2%	28.5%	

References

Barnes GK, Ray MJ, Oberman A, Kouchoukos NT (1977) Changes in working status of patients following coronary bypass surgery. JAMA 238:1259

Benesch L, Neuhaus KL, Rivas-Martin J, Loogen F (1979) Clinical results and return to work after coronary heart surgery. In: Roskamm H, Schmuzinger M (eds) Coronary heart surgery — a rehabilitation measure. Springer, Berlin Heidelberg New York, p 379

Blümchen G, Scharf-Bornhofen E, Brandt D, van den Bergh C, Bierck G (1979) Clinical results and social implications in patients after coronary bypass surgery. In: Roskamm H, Schmuzinger M (eds) Coronary heart surgery — a rehabilitation measure. Springer, Berlin Heidelberg New York, p 375

Council on Scientific Affairs (1979) Indications for aortocoronary bypass graft surgery. JAMA 242:2709

David P (1979) Contributing factors preventing return to work of cardiac surgery patients. In: Roskamm H, Schmuzinger M (eds) Coronary heart surgery — a rehabilitation measure. Springer, Berlin Heidelberg New York, p 370

Gunnar RM, Loeb HS, Bärwolf-Gohlke C, Palac RT, Piffarre R (1980) Coronary artery bypass surgery in chronic angina pectoris: Effect on symptoms and longevity. In: Mason DT (ed) Advances in heart disease. Grune & Stratton, New York (Clinical Cardiology Monographs, vol 3)

Hammermeister KE, de Routen TA, English MT, Dodge HT (1979) The effect of surgical versus medical therapy on return to work. Am J Cardiol 44:105

Kass Wenger N, Hurst JW (1980) Coronary bypass surgery as a rehabilitative procedure. Cardiac Rehabilitation Vol 11, No 3, Fall 1980

Lawrie GM, Morris GC, Howell JF, Ogura JW, Spencer WH, Cashion WR, Winters WL, Beazley HL, Chapman DW, Peterson PK, Lie JT (1979) Results of aorto-coronary bypass more than 5 years after operation in 434 patients. Am J Cardiol 40:665

Lichtlen P, Liese W, Leitz K, Borst HG (1978) Postoperative Klinik nach aorto-koronarem Venenbypass in Relation zum Ausmaß der Revaskularisation. Z. Kardiol 67:83

Niles NW, van der Salm TJ, Cutler BS (1980) Return to work after coronary artery bypass operation. J Thorax Cardiovasc Surg 79:916

Oberman A, Kouchoukos NT (1979) Working status of patients following coronary bypass surgery. Am Heart J 98:132

Rimm AA, Barboriak JJ, Anderson AJ, Simon JS (1976) Changes in occupation after aorto coronary vein-bypass operation. JAMA 236:361

Rothlin ME, Senning Å (1977) Indikationen, Risiko und Spätergebnisse der Koronarchirurgie. Internist (Berlin) 18:322

Schnellbacher K, Heidecker K, Samek L, Görnandt L, Stürzenhofecker P, Roskamm H (1980) Arbeitsfähigkeit nach aorto-koronarer Bypass-Operation bei Patienten ≤ 55 Jahre. Z Kardiol 69:220

Wallwork J, Potter B, Caves PK (1978) Return to work after coronary artery surgery for angina. Br Med J II:1680

Return to Work After Coronary Surgery: Is There a Need for a Comprehensive Rehabilitation Program?

N. Danchin, P. David, P. Robert, and M.G. Bourassa

Vocational rehabilitation in coronary patients constitutes a major concern for physicians and cardiologists. Although coronary surgery allows for a spectacular amelioration in the functional status of those patients, it does not seem to improve work resumption noticeably. The purpose of the present study was to analyze the working status of male patients during the 5 years following aortocoronary bypass surgery, and to determine factors related to postoperative return to work.

Return to work was studied by means of a questionnaire in 1287 consecutive male patients, aged less than 60 years, who had undergone aortocoronary bypass surgery at the Montreal Heart Institute between 1973 and 1978. Patients in whom valvular surgery was coupled to coronary surgery were excluded. Answers were obtained in 1234 patients (96%) and mean follow-up was 36 months (7–77 months). Mean age of the group was 50 years (28–59 years).

The first part of the study was designed to evaluate the work profile of the group after surgery. Seventy-six percent returned to work, but 20% of them stopped working later on, during the observation period; 24% never resumed work after surgery. When analyzed on a yearly basis, the percentage of patients working peaked, 2 years after surgery (66.5%), and then declined to 53%, 5 years after operation (Fig. 1); in other words, 1 in 2 patients had no occupation 5 years after surgery (approximately 10 years before the usual age of retirement).

In the second part of the study, multivariate discriminant analysis was used in order to determine which of the preoperative variables retained were correlated with the working status 1 year after surgery. The two most important parameters were (1) the duration of the preoperative period of not working, and (2) the amount of physical effort involved in the preoperative occupation. Other significant variables were presence of an associated illness, educational level, functional class of angina, duration of symptoms, age, level of income and work status of the wife.

It is particularly interesting to note that socioeconomic variables were the most decisive. Among medical variables, the data corresponding to the objective severity of coronary artery disease were not correlated with work status after surgery: previous myocardial infarction, abnormal preoperative ECG, positive stress test, number of coronary vessels diseased, ventriculogram, ejection fraction, cardiothoracic ratio, number of vessels grafted, aneurysmectomy and degree of myocardial revascularization had no influence on return to work.

In the last part of our study, we analyzed the role of postoperative health status, at the time of the survey, on return to work after surgery. Patients who judged that their health was very good had a much better return to work than those who judged that it was good or poor: 94%, 73%, and 50%, respectively. Similarly, the patients whose condition was better after coronary surgery had a good rate of return to work, whereas it was much lower in those whose condition was deteriorated, when compared to their preoperative health status (79% versus 56%). Lastly, patients who described severe chest pain (class III or IV) at the

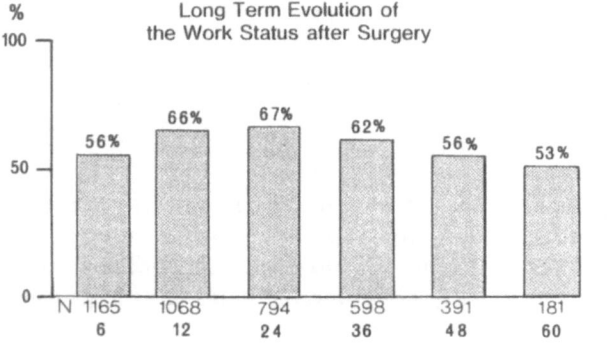

Fig. 1. Working status after coronary surgery in men under 60 years old

time of the survey had a low rate of work resumption (51%); in those with moderate (class II) or atypical chest pain the rate was 77%, and it reached 89% in those described no anginal symptoms.

Discussion

Our study has been conducted in patients who had not attended any particular rehabiliation program. The rate of reemployment after coronary surgery is disappointing; there are always fewer patients employed after surgery (maximum 67% after 2 years) than there were 6 months before surgery (69%) (Fig. 2). These results are concordant with most of those reported in the literature to date [1–8], but it is our opinion that they could be substantially enhanced. In this respect, close analysis of the factors influencing return to work after surgery should prove particularly useful, in order to determine the points that a rehabilitation team should devote its attention to: both preoperative socioeconomic factors and postoperative subjective health status are likely to have a decisive influence on work resumption. Such a team should include physicians, physiotherapists, social workers and psychologists, and the patients ought to be taken care of both before and after surgery.

Before surgery, members of the team should proceed to a complete evaluation of each patient's situation, if possible at the time coronary angiography is performed. Time interval between hemodynamic investigations and coronary surgery ought to be reduced, as much as possible, in order to reduce the length of the preoperative period of unemployment, for many patients do not return to work after coronary arteriography. Indeed, we have seen that it is the most important preoperative factor influencing return to work after surgery, and it should be considered with special care in those patients that the team would recognize as having a poor "social prognosis" (i.e., patients with heavy jobs, low level of education and/or income, associated illness, severe angina or long-lasting cardiac symptoms). At the same time, cardiologists and physiotherapists should evaluate the extent of coronary obstruction and myocardial damage, so as to determine the possibilities of exercise rehabilitation after operation.

After surgery, social workers would have to help the patients in being reengaged in their former employment or in finding more appropriate occupations — particularly, professions with a lesser physical demand. Similarly, physiotherapists with the physicians advice, would undertake the patients physical training, in order to improve their functional capacity;

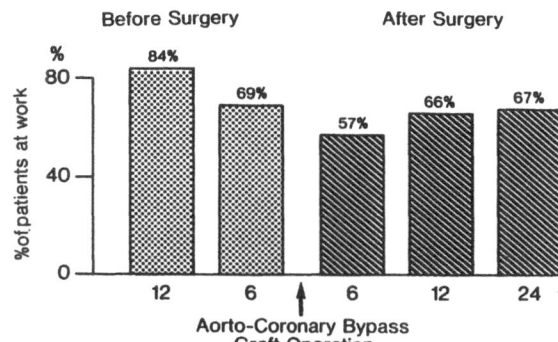

Fig. 2. Comparison of the working status before and after coronary surgery

this seems to be particularly important in patients whose subjective health status has not been notably improved after surgery and who must not feel that they are "abandoned" and beyond all medical or surgical help – we have seen, above, the importance of subjective health status after surgery on reemployment. Lastly, although the influence of psychological factors has not been analyzed in our study, we feel that psychologists should be particularly helpful in many patients, in whom open-heart surgery leads to exaggerated anxiety that impairs both their general quality of life and, consequently, their desire to return to work.

In conclusion, we think that the "social results" of coronary surgery are rather disappointing, since one out of two patients has stopped working 5 years after operation. Nevertheless, the recognition of factors having a negative influence on work resumption leads to some optimism as to the possible action of a comprehensive rehabilitation team that would take care of the patients before and in the weeks following surgery.

References

1 Barnes GK, Ray MJ, Oberman A, Kouchoukos NT (1977) Changes in working status of patients following coronary bypass surgery. JAMA 238:1259
2 Benesch L, Neuhaus KL, Rivas-Martin J, Loogen F (1979) Clinical results and return to work after coronary heart surgery. In: Roskamm H, Schmuzinger M (eds) Coronary heart surgery. A rehabilitation measure. Springer, Berlin Heidelberg New York, p 379
3 David P (1979) Contributing factors preventing return to work of cardiac surgery patients. In: Roskamm H, Schmuzinger M (eds) Coronary heart surgery. A rehabilitation measure. Springer, Berlin Heidelberg New York, p 370
4 Hammermeister KE, de Rouen TA, Englisch MT, Dodge HT (1979) Effect of surgical versus medical therapy on return to work in patients with coronary artery disease. Am J Cardiol 44:105
5 Russel RO Jr, Wayne JB, Kroenfeld J, Charles ED, Oberman A, Kouchoukos NT, White C, Rogers W, Mantle JA, Rackley CE (1980) Surgical versus medical therapy for treatment of unstable angina: Changes in work status and family income. Am J Cardiol 45:134
6 Symmes JC, Lenkei SCM, Berman ND (1978) Influence of aorto coronary bypass surgery on employment. Can Med Assoc J 118:268
7 Wallwork J, Potter B, Caves PK (1978) Return to work after coronary artery surgery for angina. Br Med J II:1680
8 Westaby S, Sapsford RN, Bentall HH (1979) Return to work and quality of life after surgery for coronary artery disease. Br Med J II:1028

Adjusting to Coronary Artery Disease: Coping with the Problems of Convalescence Following Myocardial Infarction

T.P. Hackett and N.H. Cassem

Just as delay is the principal problem of the pre-hospital period in myocardial infarction, depression is the major stress of the post-hospital period or convalescense [1, 2]. This depressive response is said to be universal. Among others, Paul Dudley White acknowledged its importance in his statement, "It is important to realize that the heart may recover more rapidly than the depressed mental state which is so often a complication" [3]. The intensity of the depression varies from patient to patient, as does its course in time. It is reactive in nature, meaning that it occurs in response to the changes of life-style the infarction brings about. Generally, depressive thoughts focus about predictable concerns such as survival, earning capacity, ability to function as a family member and parent, as a sexual partner, and to lead an active life.

Although such concerns begin to crop up in the patient's thinking on the third hospital day, seldom is the depressive reaction severe enough to make itself known to the primary physician or other caretakers. The patient usually does not appear depressed and keeps his worries to himself. Mood, in the coronary care unit, is more apt to be anxious on the first and second days and relieved by the third (Fig. 1), at which time the patient comes to realize the acute threat to his life has been reduced. As a consequence he is apt to appear more relieved and at ease than depressed.

The post infarction depression generally becomes obvious at one specific point in the natural history of this disorder. In our experience the realization of an underlying depression occurs the day the patient returns home. The specific precipitant is the sense of weakness that develops when the patient exerts himself. Usually this is experienced when the individual walks around his house for the first time or climbs a flight of stairs. For this reason we have coined the term "homecoming depression." Unless the patient has participated in an activity program while hospitalized this sense of weakness will occur. In almost every instance the individual who has not been told to expect to tire easily because of bed rest muscle atrophy, misinterprets this weaknes as a harbinger of cardiac decline. Such an interpretation causes the patient to feel that his heart is more severely damaged than he has been told or than the doctor has realized. Not infrequently, this misinterpretation is followed by the appearance of some of the criteria for depression which have been developed by the American Psychiatric Association [4]. There are eight such criteria for a major depressive episode. When five of the eight are found in a patient a depression is said to be definite; when four are present it is probable; the time limit is for 1 month or more:

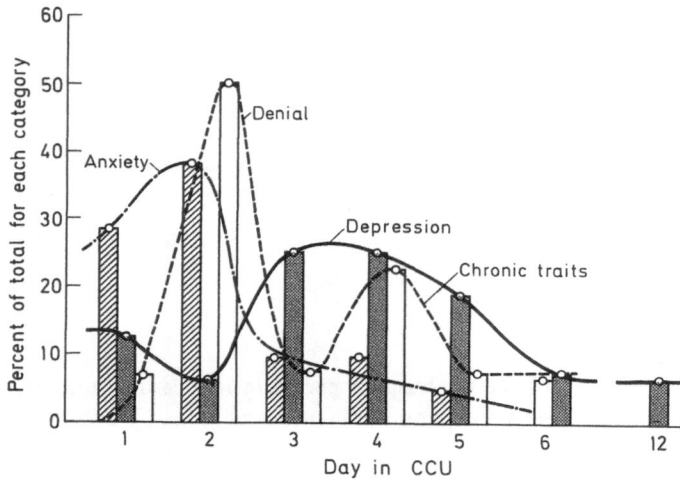

Fig. 1. Reactions in the first few days after myocardial infarction. (From Hackett TP, Cassem NH (1971) Ann Intern Med 75:9—14)

1. Sleep disturbance
2. Poor appetite — weight gain or loss
3. Fatigue — the loss of energy
4. Psychomotor agitation or retardation
5. Loss of interest in activities such as hobbies, sports — decreased libido (sex drive) along with specific sexual disturbances such as impotence or premature ejaculation
6. Decreased ability to concentrate and poor memory — sometimes to the point of "pseudo-dementia" — more prominent and worrisome in white-collar workers who depend upon cognitive skills
7. Feelings of guilt or self-reproach
8. Recurrent thoughts of death or suicide or the wish to be dead

Add to these in the case of the cardiac patient the following criteria:
9. Irritability
10. Anxiety when approaching new situations, such as driving in traffic or return to work
11. Somatic symptoms — headache, dizziness, lightheadedness

This depressive reaction we refer to as homecoming depression usually contains four to six of these criteria. It is, however, a normal or reactive depression which usually clears up in approximately 3 months. Nonetheless, while it lasts, this depressive response can be difficult for the patient to endure and a source of discouragement and sometimes despairs for the family. The duration of this depression is much longer and its depth more profound in 15% of the post infarction population and can contribute to psychological invalidism. In other countries such as Australia about 3 out of 6 individuals as reported by Allan Wynn develop psychological invalidism [5].

There are a number of factors that contribute to the depth of this depression, the largest portion of which are psychological. Although the extent of myocardial damage and consequent limitation of activeties may serve as a primary determinant of the intensity of the depressive response it is by no means that most important. Among the more important determining variables are the individual's ego strength, his family support, his social support and, especially true in blue-collar populations, his job situation. Religious faith and strength of church affiliation are also of great importance in buttressing against stress.

The purpose of this report is to discuss ways in which the individual's coping capacity, particularly the use of denial, can be used to enhance successful adaptation to the stress imposed by the homecoming depression. There are some simple ways of improving the ability to cope and some that are highly complex. As far as I know none has been tested in any scientific way and yet the majority fall within the realm of common sense.

Coping Tactics in Myocardial Infarction Convalescence

I.   Education
     A) Anticipation
     B) Explanation — "draw a heart"
        1. Demythify
        2. Sexual education
II. Activity programs
     A) Physical conditioning
     B) Planned leisure activity
     C) Relaxation — meditation — hypnosis
III. Habit modification
     A) Membership in heart club
     B) Smoking/diet groups, e.g., "smokenders"
     C) Behavior modification — type A
IV. Psychopharmacology
     A) Anxiolytics — benzodiazepines
     B) Antidepressants
        1. Tricyclic antidepressants
        2. Monoamine oxidase inhibitors
     C) Neuroleptics
V.   Denial/optimism

Education

Providing information about a patient's condition, whether it be cancer or heart disease, is one of the major ways in which we help the patient cope with the stress of his condition. While in times past it was more common to avoid providing a full explanation lest the patient be thereby rendered more frightened, this custom has long since been discarded by most physicians. The latter have now come to believe that with few exceptions knowledge protects rather than harms the patient. Proper information is a shield against fantasies and the abundance of myths and misinformation prevalent about all medical conditions, but particularly in common maladies such as heart disease and cancer. Education is largely provided to the cardiac patient by a variety of booklets and pamphlets sponsored by and published by professional societies such as the American Heart Association. Most of these publications are excellent and they cover the major aspects of cardiovascular illness. Nothing, however, is as effective an instrument of education as the personal instruction given by the physicians.

Anticipation

Anticipation, as an adjunct of education, is particularly important in reducing the incidence and intensity of homecoming depression. If the patient can be told that getting depressed is a normal aspect of recovery from a heart attack, he is apt to feel less unique and alone with his sickness. If he is informed that the sense of easy fatigue and weakness is the result of muscle atrophy secondary to bed rest and does not reflect cardiac status, the impact of this symptom is dampened considerably.

Explanation

In early convalescence we have found it useful to learn the patient's concept of what a heart attack is and how it is repaired by drawing a picture of what has happened in his heart. The picture is then used as a means of correcting misinformation and providing an accurate account of the facts. We use the drawing to lead into a discussion of the patient's notions of the limitations posed by his heart attack. This, in turn, leads into a discussion of activity programs and the importance of physical conditioning. We also advocate taking a careful sexual history which will include the patient's expectations of sexual vitality following his heart attack. The physiology of sexual intercourse is then explained with an idea of demonstrating its naturalness, desirability and low risk.

Activity Programs

Physical conditioning under close medical supervision is, to my way of thinking, one of the best ways of restoring confidence to the convalescent myocardial infarction patient. Exercise bolsters his sense of physical competence and enlarges his domain of activity. It encourages optimism and confidence. Physical conditioning stands out as an affirmation of life. There is a good deal of evidence, most of which is anecdotal and uncontrolled, that a program of physical activity does reduce the incidence of depression and restores a favorable balance of mind to the individual. As a coping tactic to ward off post infarction depression it has no peer. This is my belief. It remains to be demonstrated in a scientifically convincing way.

Habit Modification

Changing long-standing habits of eating, drinking and smoking, not to mention work and leisure, is very difficult to accomplish. There is no easy way to induce an individual to stop smoking, to eat less, work less, relax more and to exercise regularly. A variety of methods have been attempted to alter these functions including special clinics, national programs, the formation of heart clubs and the utilization of the relaxation response and autohypnosis in individual and group circumstances. Behavior modification schemes have also been employed in an attempt to alter type A behavior. Although a number of studies evaluating these modalities are currently being done, none has reported exciting results. If one examines the data on smoking cessation alone we find that all the individuals who stop smoking, 95% do so on their own, independent of any program of intervention. I suspect the same is true in other behaviors as well. This is not to say that we do not have every good reason to pursue ways to curb these harmful behaviors, but only to point out that the way to do so is difficult and probably requires a new type of approach before high success is obtained. This is an area that requires a good deal of investigation.

Psychopharmacology

The individual can be taught to cope with anxiety-provoking situations by being given anti-anxiety drugs, in particular the benzodiazapines. Antidepressants, both the tricyclic compounds and the monoamine oxidase inhibitor group have been used in the depressed post infarction patient with limited success. The use of antidepressant medication is associated with orthostatic hypotension, unpleasant anticholinergic side effects, conduction systems defects, and myocardial depression; however, as experience has widened with these compounds we have come to use them more freely in the convalescent stages of myocardial infarction when the depressive response warrants this. However, since the majority of these depressions are reactive they are not particularly responsive to any of the antidepressant medications.

Specific Coping Tactics

Most investigators agree that the defense of denial, in one form or another, is a common method of coping with serious illness [6, 7, 8]. We have defined denial as the conscious or unconscious repudiation of part or all of the total available meaning of an event to allay fear, anxiety or other unpleasant affects [6]. Specifically, the denier is someone who says that he feels no fear in the coronary care unit and that he felt no fear during the events leading up to his coming to the hospital. He is confident of survival and places full faith in the skill of his physicians. Generally he is outgoing and optimistic. Not unfrequently, this type of individual distresses his physican because he tends to minimize the extent of cardiac damage and appears to disregard the seriousness of his illness. Denial ranges all the way from the repudiation of having had a heart attack to fully admitting that a heart attack took place, but to minimizing the consequences. The majority of individuals that we have examined in the coronary care unit over the past 20 years have exhibited a sizable amount of denial. This ranges from major denial to no denial. The term major denial is used to describe persons who state unequivocally that they felt no fear at any time throughout their hospital stay or early in their lives. The designation partial denial was assigned to those who initially denied being frightened but who eventually admitted feeling at least some fear. Minimal or no denial was used to describe patients who either complained of anxiety or who readily admitted being frightened. In this group no consistent criteria for the use of denial could be found. Major denial was found in roughly 40% of the patients; partial denial in 50% and minimal denial in 10%. Sidney Croog interviewed 345 men three weeks after myocardial infarction and was told by 20% that they had not had a heart attack [9].

It came as a surprise to us initially when we discovered an inverse relationship between denial and mortality [10]. The higher the denial the more apt the patient was to survive the hospital experience. While the actual number of cases was small, this was the first inkling that denial would be protective. While we initially felt that this defense might be suitable as an emergency measure we were convinced that it would produce uncooperative individuals who would continue with an unsuitable diet and smoking, making no attempt to modify their life-style, and who, even more seriously, would not stay in touch with their physicians. Subsequently work from our group and from others has revealed that this is not the case [11, 12, 13]. Individuals who deny in general suffer less depression over time and have fewer complications. Deniers also comply with their medical regimens just as well as their non-denying counterparts. Individuals who successfully employ denial seem to do better in terms of their subjective responses, sense of well-being, and lessened depression. One would suppose from this that their physical state would also suffer less damage than that of anxious and depressed patients.

Our thinking on denial has changed considerably over the last 15 years. Whereas originally we were impressed with the way patients were able to deny fear, concern, worry, and dread — were able, so to speak, to "shelve" these unpleasant affects — more recently we have become increasingly impressed by other aspects of the dernier's mental structure. Originally, when we constructed our scale for measuring denial we tended to focus on mechanisms by which the denial of stress was achieved. Do patients minimize, displace, intellectualize, rationalize, undo? The Hackett-Cassem Denial Scale was based upon an examination and weighing of 31 items all pertaining to what the patient denied and how he denied [14]. An equally important component to the coping strategy of denial is something that is not mentioned in the scale, but has come to mean as much to us as the original notion of denying stress. This has to do with affirmation. The denier not only minimizes, reduces, or negates stress, he is also confident of his survival, optimistic of his chances for retaining his original place in society and appears fully convinced that he will regain the same degree of vitality that he had before his heart attack. Just as stress is denied, so is life and health affirmed.

One might seriously question the value of this information to the medical practitioner, particularly since it does not come to us as the result of a controlled, prospective study. Essentially, what this information suggests is that inducing a state of mind in which the patient worries less, or not at all, despite full awareness of the facts of his illness, when accompanied by optimism and full hope for the future, imparts a sense of well-being to the individual which bodes well for his physical and mental well-being. Such individuals do not suffer extended post infarction depressions; they seem to return earlier to work as well as to sexual functioning.

If denial and optimism do indeed correlate with a longer and more happy survival, then the physician, more than any other professional, is in a better position to implant and maintain the substance and structure of this vital process of adaptation.

References

1   Hackett TP, Cassem NH (1969) Factors contributing to delay in responding to the signs and symptoms of acute myocardial infarction. Am J Cardiol 24:651
2   Moss AJ, Goldstein S (1970) The pre-hospital phase of acute myocardial infarction. Circulation 41:737

3 White PD (1951) Heart disease. McMillan, New York
4 American Psychiatric Association (1980) Diagnostic criteria, DSM III, Dallas
5 Wynn A (1967) Unwarranted emotional distress in men with ischemic heart disease (IHD), Med J Aust 2:847
6 Weisman AD, Hackett TP (1961) Predilection to death: Death and dying as a psychiatric problem. Psychosom Med 23:232−257
7 Gentry WD, Foster S, Haney T (1972) Denial as a determinate of anxiety and perceived health status in the coronary care unit. Psychosom Med 34:38−44
8 Soloff PH (1978) Denial and rehabilitation of the post myocardial infarction. Int J Psychiatry Med 8:125−132
9 Croog SH, Shapiro DS, Levine S (1971) Denial among male heart patients. Psychosom Med 33:385−397
10 Hackett TP, Cassem NH, Wishnie MA (1968) The Coronary Care Unit: An appraisal of its psychological hazards. N Engl J Med 279:1365−1370
11 Soloff PH (1980) Affects of denial on mood compliance and quality of functioning after cardiovascular rehabilitation. Gen Hosp Psychiatry 2:134−140
12 Soloff PH, Bartel AG (1979) Affects of denial on mood and performance in cardivascular rehabilitation. J Chronic Dis 32:307, 313
13 Stern MJ, Pascale L, Ackermann A (1977) Life adjustment following myocardial infarction. Arch Intern Med 137:1680−1685
14 Hackett TP, Cassem NH (1974) Development of a quantitative rating scale to assess denial. J Psychosom Res 18:93−100

Evidence of a Relation Between Higher Nervous Activity and Sudden Death

A. Schöneberger, R.L. Verrier, and B. Lown

The overwhelming majority of sudden cardiac deaths occurs in patients with atherosclerotic coronary disease. However, structural lesions, such as myocardial infarction or thrombosis, are only found in a small percentage of these cases [1, 2].

The immediate mechanism of sudden death is most frequently ventricular fibrillation or ventricular tachycardia degenerating into fibrillation [3, 4].

Thus, it seems reasonable to hypothesize that impaired coronary perfusion renders the myocardium electrically unstable and that factors as yet not clearly identified precipitate the catastrophic arrhythmia in these hearts. Among these factors that could trigger ventricular fibrillation are those originating in higher nervous centers. In reviewing the evidence for such a relation we shall first consider animal models and then assess the problem in man (Table 1).

Evidence in Animals: Central Neural Effects, Sympathetic Nervous System

It has long been known that in the experimental animal sympathetic activity exerts a profound effect on cardiac rhythm. Electrical stimulation of hypothalamic areas in the brain or of the stellate ganglia increases sympathetic tone and predisposes to various arrhythmias [5,

Table 1. Animal studies examining the effects of central and peripheral nervous system and of psychologic stress on cardiac rhythm and vulnerability to ventricular fibrillation

---

Central nervous system
chemical, electrical CNS-stimulation
pharmacological interventions altering neural outflow

Peripheral nervous system
Sympathetic
stimulation of cardiac fibers
endogenous, exogenous catecholamines
surgical, pharmacological sympathectomy
sympathetic tone during myocardial ischemia

Parasympathetic
stimulation of vagal fibers
acetylcholine, metacholine
surgical, pharmalogical parasympathectomy

Sympathetic-parasympathetic interactions

Psychological stresses
vulnerability testing during nonischemic conditions
ventricular arrhythmia during myocardial ischemia

6, 7]. In the ischemic heart these interventions augment cardiac susceptibility to ventricular fibrillation [8]. Similar effects can be elicited by the administration of sympathomimetic drugs [9]. Surgical or pharmacological reduction of sympathetic activity affords protection of the heart against rhythm disturbances. Some of the new animal work is based on nerve recording studies showing that increased CNS serotonin concentration reduces central sympathetic outflow to the heart [10]. Rabinowitz and Lown studied the effect of such an inhibition of central sympathetic tone on ventricular irritability [11]. The method of measuring cardiac vulnerability consisted of electrical induction of repetitive ventricular extrasystoles (RE) which occurred reproducibly when 66% of the fibrillatory current was administered (Fig. 1) [12]. The biochemical precursors of serotonin L-tryptophan or 5-hydroxy-L-tryptophan were given to anesthetized dogs together with the monoamine oxidase inhibitor phenelzine and the selective peripheral L-amino acid decarboxylase inhibitor carbidopa. Phenelzine prevents the degradation of serotonin, and carbidopa which does not cross the blood-brain barrier inhibits formation of serotonin in the periphery but not in the brain. A sustained increase in RE threshold was only observed with administration of phenelzine and carbidopa, which increase CNS serotonin levels. A similar effect could also be shown with the infusion of the pineal hormone melatonin, which also augments serotonin concentrations in the brain [13].

Psychological Stress and Ventricular Fibrillation

Until recently no experimental data was available examining the crucial question whether behavioral and psychological variables can alter cardiac vulnerability to ventricular fibrillation. Lown and co-workers studied this problem using the method of RE testing which — as mentioned above — does not require the induction of ventricular fibrillation [14, 15]. For the psychological studies dogs were exposed to two different environments, one of which was stressful. The latter consisted of a Pavlovian sling in which the dogs received a low current shock at the end of each experimental period on 3 successive days. When put in the sling on the fourth day the dogs were restless, exhibited tremor and had an elevated heart rate. In this environment the stimulus current for RE averaged 17 ± 2 mA whereas in the nonstressful setting the mean threshold was markedly higher, amounting to 32 ± 5 mA (Fig. 2). It

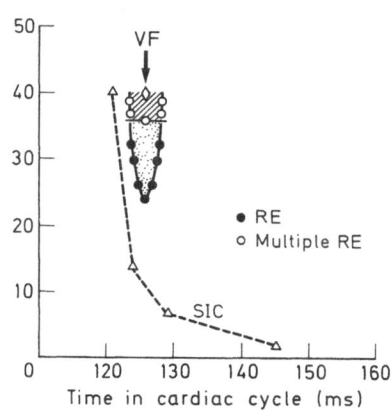

Fig. 1. Repetitive extrasystole *(RE)* and ventricular fibrillation *(VF)* threshold relation. Electrical diastole was scanned with cathodal stimuli of increasing current strength (in ma shown on the ordinate). RE threshold was consistently 66% of VF current. *SIC*, strength interval curve. Multiple REs appear before VF threshold is reached [12]

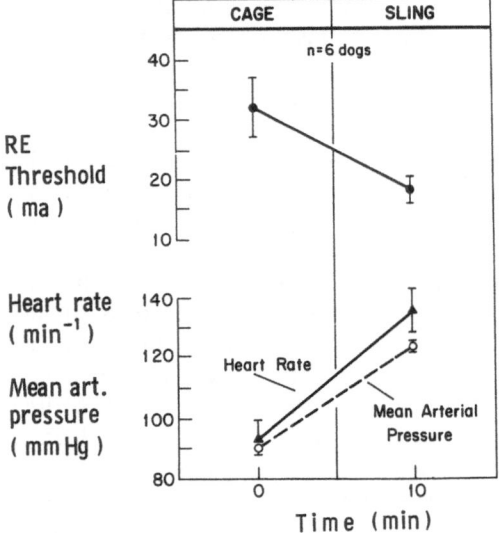

Fig. 2. Effect of the psychologically aversive sling environment and the non-aversive cage setting on repetitive extrasystole *(RE)* threshold, heart rate, and arterial pressure [15]

could also be shown that the psychologically aversive sling environment may provoke ventricular arrhythmia in the ischemic heart without electrical stimulation [16]. The animals were conditioned as described. A balloon occluder previously implanted around the left anterior descending coronary artery was inflated. After 48 h, when the animals had recovered from occlusion and were free of arrhythmia, they were reexposed to the two environments (Fig. 3). The sling setting consistently provoked serious ventricular arrhythmia, which disappeared when the animals were returned to the nonaversive cage setting.

Evidence of a Relation Between Higher Nervous Activity and Sudden Death in Man

The experimental studies presented above seem to indicate that certain psychological stresses can provoke malignant ventricular arrhythmia in the animal with myocardial ischemia. It is much more difficult to show such a direct relationship between neural and psychologic factors and sudden death in man. Thus, we shall first consider the effect of higher nervous activity on ventricular arrhythmia and then its possible role in sudden death (Table 2).

Psychological Stress and Ventricular Arrhythmia

For centuries physicians have been aware of the effects of psychologic factors on heart rhythm. It has been objectively shown that such stressful situations as speaking in public, automobile driving, and spectator sports can provoke ventricular ectopy in normal humans and in those with coronary heart disease [17, 18]. Lown and De Silva demonstrated that standardized psychologic stresses can evoke advanced grades of VPBs in patients with high grade ventricular arrhythmias [19] (Fig. 4). Similarly a marked increase of the frequency of VPBs was observed in a patient who witnessed a discussion of her condition by the chief of service during rounds in the intensive care unit (Fig. 5).

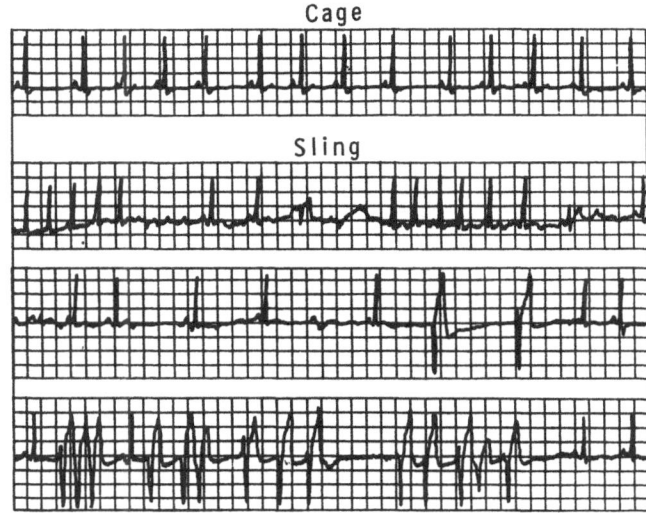

Fig. 3. Psychologic stress provokes ventricular ectopy *(VE)* in the awake dog during experimental myocardial infarction. In the nonstressful environment of the cage there is no VE. In the stressful sling setting VE appears [16]

Psychological Factors and Sudden Death

It is widely believed that emotions may predispose to sudden cardiac death. Engel has provided a collection of anecdotal reports relating the occurrence of sudden death to intense emotions such as grief, fear, frustration, rage, and joy [20]. Epidemiological studies indicate an increased prevalence of sudden death during bereavement and following significant life changes [21, 22]. In the first 6 months of loss of a spouse, the death rate among widows and widowers 55 years of age or older increased 40% above the expected rate for a married population matched for age [21].

Table 2. Studies in humans examining the effects of neural activity on ventricular arrythmia and of psychological factors in sudden death

---

Neural activity and ventricular arrythmia
infusion of catecholamines or cholinergic drugs
arrythmia during sleeping-waking cycle
stressful situations in coronary heart disease
standardized psychological stress tests
testing of the autonomic nervous system

Psychological factors and ventricular fibrillation
epidemiology of mortality in coronary heart disease
single case reports of cause and effect relation
the biologic model of the long Q-T syndrom

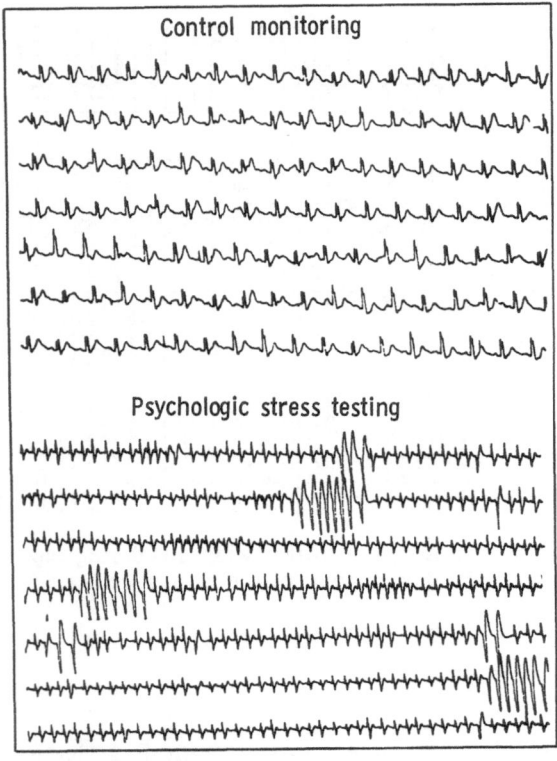

Fig. 4. High grade of ventricular ectopy *(VE)* induced by psychologic stress testing. Top tracing represents monitor lead before testing. Bottom tracing shows supraventricular tachycardia and high grade VE during psychologic stress [19]

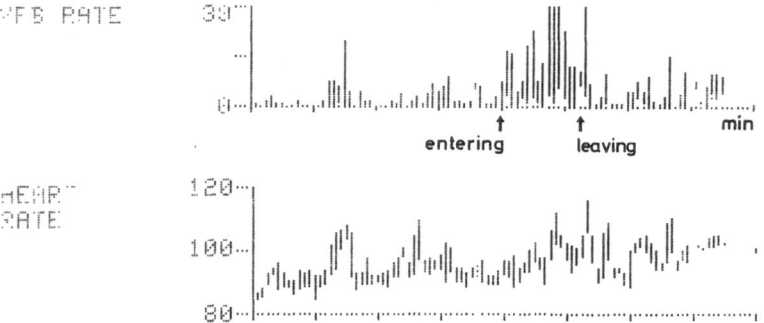

Fig. 5. Rate of ventricular premature beats (VPB/min) in a patient in the intensive care unit. Number of VPBs increases during rounds of the chief of service and discussion of the patient's poor prognosis. Lower panel shows heart rate/min

A study by Weinblatt and co-workers found that a low level of education increased the risk of sudden death in men with complex VPBs after myocardial infarction [23]. It was speculated that the psychosocial stresses in such a setting may provoke a different pattern of autonomic nervous system output in relation to educational background.

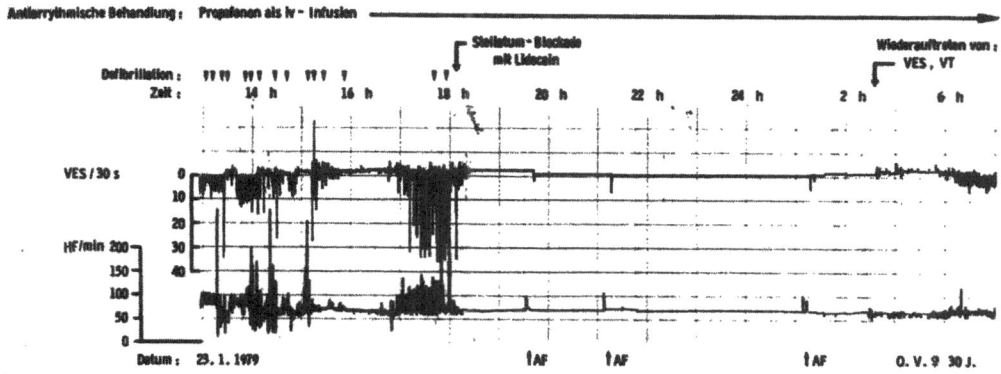

Fig. 6. Trend recording of frequency of ventricular premature beats (VES/30s) and heart rate (HF/min) in a female patient with the latent long Q-T syndrome. Defibrillation was required several times from 1 pm til 6 pm (18h) before blockade of the left stellate ganglion abolished ventricular ectopy and fibrillation. VES reappeared later. The antiarrhythmic agent propafenon was administered intravenously. *AF*, artifact [29]

However, except in individual cases — as reported by Wellens et al. [24] and Lown et al. [25] — it is difficult to establish the direct evidence demonstrating a cause-effect relationship between psychologic factors and sudden death. The most suggestive model that neural factors can be associated with the occurrence of sudden death is presented by the prolonged QT syndrome. Data from Schwartz [26] and others [27, 28] indicate that an imbalance of cardiac sympathetic innervation is responsible for the life-threatening ventricular arrhythmia frequently elicited by stress situations. Beta-adrenergic receptor blockers and ablation of the left stellate ganglion may prevent the recurrence of rhythm disturbances. A manipulation of the stellate ganglion might even in the rare patient with the latent QT syndrome (i.e., recurrent malignant ventricular arrhythmia, but no QT prolongation) be lifesaving when antiarrhythmic agents, including beta-receptor blockade, fail. Such a patient (Fig. 6) without recognizeable heart disease had many episodes of malignant ventricular arrhythmia initiated by early VPBs and underwent electrical defibrillation 99 times until blockade of the left stellate ganglion suppressed the arrhythmia. The patient then underwent surgical stellectomy and has not had recurrence of syncope or ventricular tachyarrhythmia for a follow-up period of 2 years [29].

Conclusion

The studies cited support the view that higher nervous activity may constitute a transient risk factor for sudden death. A major role can be ascribed to the sympathetic limb of the autonomic nervous system. Recent advances in neurochemistry and psychopharmacology promise profound new insights into the interaction between brain and heart.

References

1 Roberts WC (1972) Relationship between coronary thrombosis and myocardial infarction. Mod Concepts Cardiovasc Dis 41:7
2 Reichenback DD, Moss NS, Meyer E (1977) Pathology of the heart in sudden coronary death. Am J Cardiol 39:865
3 Pantridge JR, Geddes JS (1967) A mobile intensive care unit in the management of moycardial infarction. Lancet II:271
4 Liberthson RR, Nagel EL, Hirschman JC, Nussenfeld SR (1974) Prehospital ventricular defibrillation: Prognosis and follow-up course. N Engl J Med 291:317
5 Korteweg GCJ, Boeles TF, Tencate J (1957) Influence of stimulation of some subcortical areas on electrocardiogram. J Neurophysiol 20:100
6 Verrier RL, Calvert A, Lown B (1975) Effect of posterior hypothalamic stimulation on the ventricular fibrillation threshold. Am J Physiol 228:923
7 Han J, Garcia de Jalon P, Moe G (1964) Adrenergic effects on cardiac vulnerability. Circ Res 14:516
8 Satinsky J, Kosowsky B, Lown B, Kerzner J (1971) Ventricular fibrillation induced by hypothalamic stimulation during coronary occlusion. Circulation 44:II−60
9 Rabinowitz SH, Verrier RL, Lown B (1976) Muscarinic effect of vagosympathetic trunk stimulation on the repetitve extrasystole threshold. Circulation 53:622
10 Baum T, Shropshire AT (1975) Inhibition of efferent sympathetic nerve activity by 5-hydroxytryptamine. Neuropharmacology 14:227
11 Rabinowitz SH, Lown B (1978) Central neurochemical factors related to serotonin metabolism and cardiac vulnerability for repetitive electrical activity. Am J Cardiol 41:516
12 Matta RJ, Verrier RL, Lown B (1976) The repetitive extrasystole as an index of vulnerability to ventricular fibrillation. Am J Physiol 230:1469
13 Blatt CM, Rabinowitz SH, Lown B (1977) The effect of melatonin on repetitive ventricular activity in the dog. Circulation 56:III−237
14 Lown B, Verrier RL, Corbalan R (1973) Psychologic stress and threshold for repetitive ventricular response. Science 182:834
15 De Silva RA, Verrier RL, Lown B (1978) The effect of psychological stress and vagal stimulation with morphine on vulnerability to ventricular fibrillation in the conscious dog. Am Heart J 95:197
16 Corbalan R, Verrier RL, Lown B (1974) Psychological stress and ventricular arrhythmias during myocardial infarction in the conscious dog. Am J Cardiol 34:692
17 Taggart P, Gibbons D, Somerville W (1969) Some effects of motor-car driving on the normal and abnormal heart. Br Med J 4:130
18 Taggart P, Carruthers M, Somerville W (1973) Electrocardiogram, plasma catecholamines and lipids, and their modification by oxprenolol when speaking before an audience. Lancet II:341
19 Lown B, de Silva RA (1978) Roles of psychologic stress and autonomic nervous system changes in provocation of ventricular premature complexes. Am J Cardiol 41:979
20 Engel GL (1971) Sudden and rapid death during psychologic stress. Folklore or folk wisdom. Ann Intern Med 74:771
21 Parkes CM, Benjamin B, Fitzgerald R (1969) Broken heart: Statistical study of increased mortality among widowers. Br Med J I:740
22 Rahe RH, Romo M, Bennett L, Siltanen P (1974) Recent life changes, myocardial infarction and abrupt coronary death. Studies in Helsinki. Arch Intern Med 133:221
23 Weinblatt E, Ruberman W, Goldberg JD, Frank CW, Shapiro S, Chaudhary BS (1978) Relation of education to sudden death after myocardial infarction. N Engl J Med 299:60
24 Wellens HJJ, Vermeulen A, Durrer D (1972) Ventricular fibrillation occuring on arousal from sleep by auditory stimuli. Circulation 46:661

25 Lown B, Temte JV, Reich P, Gaughan C, Regestein Q, Hai H (1976) Basis for recurring ventricular fibrillation in the absence of coronary heart disease and its management. N Engl J Med 294:623

26 Schwartz PJ, Periti M, Malliani A (1975) The long Q-T syndrome. Am Heart J 89:378

27 Schwartz PJ (1978) Experimental reproduction of the long Q-T syndrome. Am J Cardiol 33:174

28 Vincent GM, Abildskov JA, Burgess MJ, Millar K (1974) Anatomic manipulation in the inherited long Q-T recurrent syncope syndrome. Am J Cardiol 33:174

29 Schoeneberger A, Bamberg E, Bussmann WD (1981) The long Q-T syndrome without Q-T prolongation. Klin Wochenschr 59:281

Incidence of Ventricular Arrhythmias in Coronary Artery Disease During Holter Monitoring and Stress Testing

H. Rüddel, B. Krug, G. Schilling, and H. Simon

Ventricular arrhythmias have been found to be associated with an increased risk of sudden death in patients with Ischemic Heart Disease (IHD) [4, 9, 12]. In these patients ventricular arrhythmias have been shown to increase with age, severity of IHD, and other clinical characteristics of advanced myocardial disease. Most studies reporting a connection between arrhythmia and emotion have been individual case studies. Some of them have employed interview procedures to elicit arrhythmias. In almost all cases the emotional events precipitating the arrhythmias are related to unpleasant life situations [7]. The occurrence of arrhythmias is higher at times when social interaction is taking place than when a patient is at rest [16]. Increased ectopic activity is associated with sexual activity and various interpersonal and work-related situations [2].

Systematic studies of the type of psychological derangement which may contribute to the formation of ventricular arrhythmia are lacking. Lown et al. [5] have demonstrated in animal studies that alterations induced by central nervous stimulation are mediated by sympathetic neural pathways to the heart and that in the intact animal vagal tone adapts to alterations in sympathetic discharge thereby modulating cardiac vulnerability. The R/S pulsing technique is commonly used to demonstrate electrical instability [17].

In animal models manipulation of the sympathetic neural input affects cardiac vulnerability. In the ischemic myocardium, such a manipulation may be a sufficient stimulus to induce fibrillation. In humans there are observations suggesting that an enhanced sympathetic activity may induce ventricular ectopic activity, but convincing date are lacking [4].

There is no specific psychological trait or behavioral pattern in patients with ventricular arrhythmias. Orth-Gomer could only find a high depresssion score (one scale in the Emotions Profile Index) as an independent factor for ventricular arrhythmias — but only in healthy men, not in men with overt CHD or risk indicators of IHD. In these two groups of patients ventricular ectopics are able to be observed more frequently and are more dangerous than in healthy controls [8]. Generally, ventricular arrhythmias are related to increasing age, hypertension, and cardiac enlargement.

The objective of the present study was to compare the yield and type of ectopic activity resulting from mental stress testing and a psychological high challenge interview situation in the laboratory, to that observed during electrocardiographic monitoring (Holter) in daily life situations over a period of 24 h.

Patients and Methods

The study population consisted of 28 male patients referred for diagnostic coronary arteriography during the period June 1979 to March 1980. Only patients in whom the diagnosis of CHD had been made on the basis of clinical history were included and all had clinically significant occlusion in one of the three major vessels. They showed at least a stenosis of 50% decrease in luminal diameter. Selective coronary arteriography was done with the

Judkins technique and cineangiograms were interpreted by experiences cardiologists and radiologists.

There was no myocardial infarction in the last 3 months prior to the examination. Except for nitrates, medication was stopped 3 to 4 days before the testing procedure began.

All patients were monitored as outpatients in their daily life situation with 24-h pertinent ECG registration prior to clinical admission. Registration and evaluation were performed with ICR equipment and VES (ventricular extrasystoles) were evaluated after the criteria described by Lown. Twenty two patients did not show rhythm abnormalities (group 1: Lown 0–1). In six patients severe VES were recorded (group 2: Lown ≥ 3). The two groups did not differ in age (group 1: $\bar{x}$ = 48 years; 35–66 years, group 2: $\bar{x}$ = 53 years; 35–58 years).

An exercise test was performed in 21 patients. The remaining seven of the study population had to be excluded from physical exercise testing because of resting angina, severe ECG alterations, or high blood pressure. We had chosen a submaximal work load ergometry in a half supine position. ECG was continously monitored and recorded on a chart recorder; blood pressure was recorded every minute by a cuff method.

As an emotional stress test, mental arithmetic under noise was chosen as a well standardized procedure [14]. During mental and psychological stress testing all patients were examined in an isolated enclosure at the same time of the day, while seated in a reclining chair. Blood pressure was recorded every minute by an ultrasonic Doppler System, heart rate continuously by ECG monitoring. In an adjacent room all data was registered on a polygraph. The evaluation and statistical analysis is only descriptive because of sample size.

Coronary-prone behavior, as described by Friedman and Rosenman [11] with the characteristics of competitive achievement, striving, aggression and hostility, and an exaggerated sense of time urgency, is assessed by the standardized stress interview, developed by Rosenman et al. [11]. This interview is a rather high challenge psychological stress test and relies on the overt behavioral style of the patient's responses and the content of his/her answer. The German version of the Type A interview has been introduced by Langosch, Rüddel and Schmidt [3, 13].

Results

In group 1 there was no pathologic ectopic ventricular arrhythmia (Lown 0–1) during continuous ECG recording (Holter) in daily life situations. In this group of 22 patients there were five with a three-vessel disease, seven with coronary artery occlusion in two vessels and ten with coronary occlusion in one artery. Sixteen patients had asynergies in the levocardiogram. During mental stress testing (N = 22) and during type A interview (N = 8) there was only one patient in whom the rate of ventricular arrhythmias increased compared to the resting condition (Table 1).

In group 2 (N = 6) all had ventricular arrhythmia (Lown ≥ 3) in Holter ECG. In coronary angiography a stenosis in three vessels was found in four patients, in two vessels in one patient and in one vessel in another patient. Four patients had asynergies in the levocardiogram (Table 1).

During mental stress testing the rate of VES increased in five of the six patients from baseline 4.5 VES/h to 30 VES/h during stress testing, but only in two patients did we find the same kind of ventricular ectopic activity compared to the monitoring during daily life situa-

Table 1

	Group 1 (N = 22)		Group 2 (N = 6)	
Holter ECG				
Lown 0	10		–	
Lown 1	12		–	
Lown 3	–		2	
Lown 4 a	–		–	
Coronary arteriography				
one-vessel disease	10		1	
two-vessel disease	7		1	
three-vessel disease	5		4	
Levocardiography				
hypokinesia	6		2	
akinesia	1		1	
aneurysm	6		1	
Exercise testing (ergometry)				
pathologic extopic activity	0	(N = 18)	0	(N = 3)
Mental stress testing				
pathologic ectopic activity	1	(N = 22)	5	(N = 6)
Type-A interview				
pathologic ectopic activity	1	(N = 8)	2	(N = 3)

Pathological findings in the two groups
Group 1 – pts without pathological ventricular arrhythmia
Group 2 – pts with high grade ventricular arrhythmia

tions with Holter ECG; four patients did not show the ventricular arrhythmias as documented by continuous ECG registration (Holter).

Discussion

Under mental stress testing and during type A interview pathologic ectopic activity could be observed in those patients who had more and more dangerous ventricular arrhythmias (Lown > 3) during continuous 24-h ECG registration. All of these patients with Lown 4a in the Holter ECG showed the same ventricular arrhythmias during mental and psychosocial stress testing in the laboratory as during daily life situations. All of these patients had a more advanced IHD. This is in keeping with the literature which states that ventricular arrhythmias do increase with increasing severity of IHD, above all with ventricular asynergy. Probably, the enhanced sympathetic activity during mental stress testing induces ventricular arrhythmias in a compromised ventricle.

The increased central nervous system activation during stress testing in the laboratory does not fully explain the differences in ectopic activity in our population, as the patients reacted in a different way concerning their arrhythmias, while the blood pressure response did not differ between patients in group 1 and in group 2.

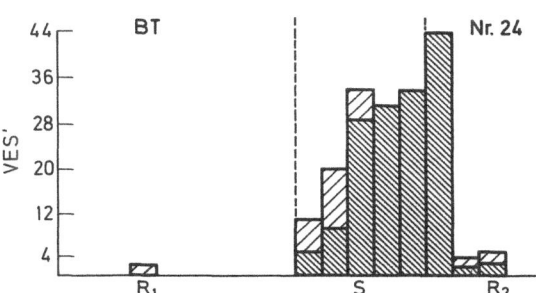

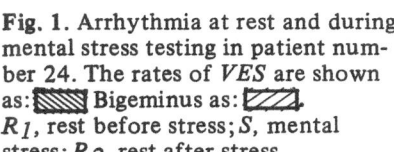

Fig. 1. Arrhythmia at rest and during mental stress testing in patient number 24. The rates of *VES* are shown as: ▨ Bigeminus as: ▨. R_1, rest before stress; S, mental stress; R_2, rest after stress

Physical exercise testing did not provoke ectopic activity in our population as seven patients out of 28 could not be exposed to ergometry. It was impossible to compare arrhythmia during mental and physical stress testing in both patient groups.

In some individual cases it could be easily demonstrated that mental stress testing could be a way of determining the electrical stability of the heart. In one instance a patient with only mild arrhythmias after myocardial infarction increased his rate of VES to 121 in the 5-min testing period (Lown 4 a).

Two weeks after this laboratory examination he suffered from severe arrhythmias (Lown 4 b) which could not be treated satisfactorily.

The combination of a compromised ventricle with an enhanced sympathetic activity can explain some findings reported in the literature. Sommerville et al., for example, observed 23 healthy persons and seven patients during public speaking. They registered more than 6 VES/h in only six of the 23 healthy Ss. but in five of the seven patients [15].

In conclusion, continuous ECG monitoring during daily life situations seems to be a better predictor of ectopic activity than physical or mental exercise testing in the laboratory, a finding that corresponds to the results reported by Lown [6].

References

1 Glass DC (1977) Behavior patterns, stress, and coronary disease. Sydnex, New York Toronto Londong

2 Hellerstein HK, Friedman EH (1970) Sexual activity and the postcoronary patient. Arch Intern Med 125:987

3 Langosch W, Rüddel H, Schmidt TH (to be published) Durchführung und Auswertung des Typ A Interviews. Münch Med Wschr

4 Lown B, Calvert AF, Armington R, Ryan M (1975) Monitoring for serious arrymias and high risk of sudden death. Circulation Suppl III, 51, 52:189

5 Lown B, Verrier RL (1976) Neural activity and ventricular fibrillation. N Engl J Med 294:1165

6 Lown B, De Silva RA (1978) Roles of psychological stress and autonomic nervous system in provocation of ventricular premature complexes. Am J Cardiol 41:979

7 Lynch JJ, Paskewitz DA, Gimbel KS, Thomas SA (1977) Psychological aspects of cardiac arrythmia. Am Heart J 93:645

8 Orth-Gomér K, Edwardo ME, Erhardt L, Sjögren A, Theorell T (1979) Relation between ventricular arrhythmias and psychological profile. In: Orth-Gomer K (ed) Studies on ischemic heart disease. Psychosocial risk indicators and ventricular arrhythmias. Stockholm

 9 Orth-Gomér K (1979) Ventricular arrhythmias and risk indicators of ischemic heart disease. In: Orth-Gomer K (ed) Studies on ischemic heart disease. Psychosocial risk indicators and ventricular arrhythmias. Stockholm

10 Rehnqvist N (1978) Ventricular arrhythmias after an acute myocardial infarction. Prognostic weight and natural history. Eur J Cardiol 7:169

11 Rosenmann RH, Friedman M, Straus R, Wurm M, Kositchek R, Hahn W, Werthessen NT (1964) A predictive study of coronary heart disease. JAMA 189:103

12 Ruberman W, Weinblatt E, Goldberg JD, Frank LW, Shapiro S (1977) Ventricular premature beats and mortality after myocardial infarction. N Engl J Med 287:750

13 Rüddel H, Langosch W, Schmidt TH, Brodner G, Neus H (to be published) Ist das Typ A Verhalten spezifisch für den Herzinfarkt? Münch Med Wschr

14 Schulte W, Neus H (1979) Bedeutung von Streßreaktionen in der Hypertoniediagnostik. Herz/Kreislauf 11:542

15 Sommerville W, Taggart P, Carruther M (1971) Addressing a medical meeting: Effect on heart rate, electrocardiogram, plasma catecholamines, free fatty acids, and triglycerides. Br Heart J 33:608

16 Thomas SA, Lynch JJ, Mills ME (1975) Psychosocial influence on heart arrhythmia in a coronary care patient. Heart Lung 4:746

17 Thompson PL, Lown B (1972) Sequential R/T pacing to expose electrical instability in the ischemic ventricle. Clin Res 20:401

Is the Influence Social Classes in Rehabilitation of Cardiac Patients Inevitable?

G. Blümchen

My answer to the question is: Yes, the influences of social classes are inevitable [1]. The following results will support this hypothesis. It is difficult to compare the influence of social classes on rehabilitation of cardiac patients in completely different societies. But it seems possible, although difficult, to compare the influence of social classes on cardiac rehabilitation between different *western* countries. The medical system in Germany is different from that of the United States and other western countries. Approximately 90% of the German population are insured by government policy. The medical insurance system is subdivided into blue-collar workers and white-collar workers. Ten percent of the population are insured privately, mainly professionals like laywers, architects, docters, teachers. Thus German society is clearly subdivided into blue-collar workers, white-collar workers and privately insured. This allows us to study the influence of social classes on rehabilitation after myocardial infarction. Therefore I will present predominantly German data.

Table 1 shows the return-to-work rate in myocardial infarctions in relation to social classes according to three German authors [2–4] and one American author [5]. The return-to-work rate after myocardial infarction increased from manual workers to "brain-workers" and was higher in the American report than in the three German ones.

Table 2 shows the return-to-work rate in patients after aortocoronary bypass operation in relation to social classes of three German authors [6–8] and one Canadian author [9]. The

Table 1. The return-to-work rate in different social classes after myocardial infarction in selected reports of three German authors and one American author

	Blue collar (%)	White collar (%)	Professionals (%)
Blümchen et al. 1978 (n = 128, t = 1.6 years)	36	–	68
Buchwalsky et al. 1980 (n = 536, t = 4 years)	–	73	
Samek et al. 1981 (n = 658, 40 y, t = 3.5 years)	67	81	
Croog, 1978, USA (n = ?, t = 1 year)	75	98	

Table 2. The return-to-work rate in different social classes after aortocoronary bypass operation in selected reports of three German authors and one Canadian author

	Blue collar (%)	White collar (%)	Professionals (%)
Gleichmann et al. 1977 (n = 64)	29	37	75
Benesch et al. 1979 (n = 191)	21	57	78
Blümchen et al. 1979 (n = 314)	27	55	43
David, 1979, Quebec (n = 908)	59	83	

return-to-work rate after bypass increased from manual workers to "brain workers" and was higher in the Canadian report than in the three German ones.

In summary, the rate of patients returning to work is partly determined by medical results, by the age of patients, the time of unemployment before the operation, and by the degree of revascularization. The long-term social outcome after myocardial infarction and after bypass operation is not determined by medical results only. Good exercise tolerance and marked improvement of symptoms months after myocardial infarction and after aorto-coronary bypass surgery are no guarantee of a high return-to-work rate.

The main determinants for the long-term social fate of conservatively treated or operated patients are our medical insurance system and especially, the motivation of the patients. The patient's decision to return to work appears to be an individual one, relating more to his perception of health and satisfaction with his employment than to his physical ability to continue working. This is especially true for patients performing heavy work.

References

1 Rose G, Marmot MG (1981) Social classes and coronary heart disease. Br Heart J 45:13
2 Blümchen G, Barthel W, van den Bergh C, Bierck G, Brandt D, Scharf-Bornhofen E, Reidemeister JC (1980) Soziales Schicksal bei operierten und konservativ behandelten Koronar- und Aneurysmapatienten. Z Kardiol 69:632
3 Buchwalsky R, Kauderer M, Tanczos P (1980) Läßt die Einschwemmkatheterunter-suchung nach Herzinfarkt prognostische Aussagen zu? Herbsttagung der Deutschen Gesellschaft für Kreislaufforschung, Münster, 2.–4.10.1980. (Vortrag Nr. 92)
4 Samek L, Spinder M, Müller F, Betz P, Schnellbacher K (1981) Vocationalrehabilitation in postinfarction patients under age 40. In: International symposium: Myocardial infarction and young age. Bad Krozingen, 30.–31.1.1981
5 Croog SH (1978) Social aspects of rehabilitation after myocardial infarction: A selective review. In: Wenger NK, Hellerstein HK (eds) Rehabilitation of the coronary patient. Wiley & Sons, New York
6 Gleichmann U, Fassbender D (1977) Probleme der Früh- und Spätrehabilitation nach Herzinfarkt. In: Schettler G, Horsch A, Mörl H, Orth H, Weizel A (eds) Der Herzinfarkt. Schattauer, Stuttgart New York

7 Blümchen G, Scharf-Bornhofen E, Brandt D, van den Bergh C, Bierck G (1979) Clinical results and social implications in patients after coronary bypass surgery. In: Roskamm H, Schmutzinger M (eds) Coronary heart surgery. Springer, Berlin Heidelberg New York
8 Benesch L, Neuhaus KL, Rivas-Martin J, Loogen F (1979) Clinical results and return to work after coronary heart surgery. In: Roskamm H, Schmutzinger M (eds) Coronary heart surgery. Springer, Berlin Heidelberg New York
9 David P (1979) Contributing factors preventing return to work of cardiac surgery patients. In: Roskamm H, Schmutzinger M (eds) Coronary heart surgery. Springer, Berlin Heidelberg New York

Patient and Family Education and Counseling: A Requisite Component of Cardiac Rehabilitation

N.K. Wenger

Goal and Rationale

The goal of patient and family education and counseling is to provide enough information about coronary disease and its management to enable the involved individuals to assume some responsiblity for their subsequent health care. An educational program is ideally instituted during the acute care hospitalization for myocardial infarction or other acute coronary episode and continued in the office of the private physician or in a hospital or community clinic or comparable facility; in the United States, many education and counseling programs are offered by voluntary health agencies. In general, a physician or a committee of physicians assumes responsibility for the content of an educational program, and periodically reviews the information presented and the recommendations for care to assure that they remain timely and appropriate. Both the actual teaching and the development of teaching materials are often best accomplished by various other health professionals – nurses, dietitians, physical or occupational therapists, social workers, etc., all of whom are able to spend more time with the patient than the physician can, particularly during the acute care hospitalization.

Because an episode of myocardial infarction constitutes a life crisis for both the patient and the family, it creates an obvious motivation for learning. Also, in the hospital setting, the variety of health professionals available can readily implement an educational program. However, if the benefits of the information presented during the hospitalization are to be maintained – because the content typically requires considerable subsequent repetition – the recommendations for care and their implementation must be reinforced on an ambulatory basis to ensure that patients have an adequate comprehension of and realistic attitude toward their cardiac problem.

Dr. Lawrence Weed (Weed 1974), well known as the advocate of the problem-oriented medical record, wisely observed that "The most powerful of all medical and paramedical personnel is the patient – highly motivated, not costing anything – even willing to pay – and there is one for every member of the population." Education for patients must be designed to provide information, motivation, and skills for this valuable member of the health care team.

Program Components

During the days in the coronary or intensive care unit fear, pain, anxiety, and fatigue impair both the physical and the mental readiness for learning. Only very simple facts should be presented and in a brief manner, typically in response to patient questions or concerns. Although much of this information may not be obtained or remembered, it relieves some uncertainties and provides the needed and timely reassurance to both the patient and the family. The general areas of emphasis include a brief explanation of the diagnosis (myocardial infarction), as well as the reasons for the safety features relative to the regulations, procedures and equipment in the coronary care unit. Once the patient and family are made aware of these considerations, they are less likely to misinterpret staff actions or comments; the reassurance offered by these explanations helps the patient adjust to a life-threatening situation. However, on occasion, educational efforts per se may provoke anxiety; for the patient coping with the emotional stress of acute infarction by denial, the presentation of information about the illness may engender additional stress. Should this become apparent, teaching may have to be deferred (Wallace and Wallace 1977). The temporary nature of most restrictions should be emphasized, identifying that, as the patient recovers and is moved to a general care area, the decrease in surveillance and in the intensity of care reflects the progress and improvement. A realistically positive attitude of all staff members is important in transmitting both to the patient and to the family their confidence initially that the patient will survive and subsequently that there is considerable likelihood of the patient's resuming a normal or near normal lifestyle.

During the remainder of the hospitalization, once the patient is relatively free of pain, has less anxiety about immediate survival, and becomes concerned with planning for return home, more detailed educational and counseling efforts are appropriate. In-hospital educational efforts which conform to the patients' perceived needs for information decrease their feelings of helpnessness in dealing with their cardiac problem, aid in restoring self-esteem after an illness which often mars their self-image, increase confidence in a successful outcome of the acute episode, and enhance the ability of individuals to cope with the problems of illness; patients acquire a sense of control and mastery over their threatening disease. These are the aims of the content components of a well-designed teaching and counseling program.

For the educational program to be successful in helping patients understand coronary disease and its manifestations, a brief review must be presented first of normal cardiac function and then of the atherosclerotic process leading to coronary obstruction. The changes that occur with myocardial infarction should be described, emphasizing the healing process. Without this background, most patients (but particularly the blue-collar workers) (Hackett 1976) are unlikely to appreciate how the pain they experienced and the disturbances of rhythm or pump function which produced symptoms could be due to atherosclerotic obstruction of the coronary arteries. This information provides the basis for the subsequent recommendations for care including coronary risk factor modification; medical therapy, including prescriptive exercise; and/or surgical intervention. Additionally, a variety of prevalent myths regarding the precipitation of myocardial infarction must be dispelled; patients not uncommonly attribute their infarction to excessive work or worry, excessive stress, a specific preinfarction high-level activity task, being excessively pressured by others, excessive alcohol use, straying from religious precepts, etc. (Goble 1969). Many adverse psychosocial outcomes after myocardial infarction or other acute coronary episode or following coronary bypass surgery appear related to the patients' perception of their health status; this component may be favorably altered by appropriate educational/informational intervention and counseling.

Since most recommendations for patient management after myocardial infarction entail a modification of habit or lifestyle, the education and counseling should provide insight into behavior patterns that may increase the risk of reinfarction or coronary death and into the value of altering these habits (Table 1). Thus the rationale for dietary changes – calorie, fat, sodium, etc., restriction – should be presented, accompanied by practical suggestions

Table 1. Educational program components for the patient with myocardial infarction. For each item listed, the date of teaching and instructor's name are recorded, as is the need for further patient education on that topic and the instructor's comments regarding the patient's comprehension (From: Wenger NK (1981) Rehabilitation of the patient with symptomatic coronary atherosclerotic heart disease. In: The Heart, 5th edn. Hurst JW (ed). Mc-Graw-Hill, New York, p 1155)

I.   Adjustment to coronary care unit
    A. Purpose of coronary care unit
    B. Regulations of unit (visiting, smoking, flowers)
    C. Monitor (sounds and leads)
    D. Intravenous infusions and medications
    E. Oxygen
    F. Activity (leg exercise, etc.)
    G. ECG, blood tests, x-rays
    H. Diet
    I. Personal emergencies (e.g. financial, job)
II. Adjustment to transfer from unit
    A. Constant observation no longer necessary
    B. Activity as prescribed
III. Information needed for adaptation to disease
    A. Normal anatomy and function of heart
    B. Development of coronary atherosclerotic heart disease
    C. Heart attack
        1. Risk factors
            (a) General discussion
            (b) Emphasis on risk factors of individual patient
        2. Warning signs of heart attack
        3. Healing-relation to physical activity
    D. Personal response to myocardial infarction
        1. Group discussion
        2. Individual conference with patient, family
IV. Plans for care after discharge from hospital
    A. Diet
        1. Group discussion
        2. Individual conference with patient, family
    B. Discharge medications (each medication,
       its dosage, is listed for teaching to patient)
    C. Activity
        1. General
        2. Sexual
        3. Work-simplification
    D. Symptoms which should be reported
    E. Rehabilitation exercises
    F. Clinic or physician appointments
    G. Community resources
V.   Other areas for teaching (e.g. pacemaker, diabetes)
VI. Educational materials given to patient (a basic pamphlet list
    checked and additional educational materials are recorded)
VII. Outpatient (clinic) education
    A. Review of IV in class and individual instruction
    B. Patient self-learning tapes and slide-tapes

for implementing these changes. The development of a reasonable diet for a patient involves consideration of that individual's food preferences and eating habits; adherence to a diet tends to be more successful when it includes enough familiar foods to encourage compliance. Further dietary adherence is enabled by providing guidelines to the patient and family for food purchasing, food preparation, and for restaurant eating. The most important individual to be educated about the recommended dietary modifications is the family member responsible for food preparation.

Cessation of cigarette smoking should be recommended and discussed both with the patients who smoke and with the members of their family. The emphasis should identify that continued smoking following myocardial infarction increasingly is associated with an excessive risk of reinfarction and cardiac death (Mulcahy et al. 1975; Wilhelmsson et al. 1975; Salonen 1980). Referral should be made to a hospital or community program to aid in smoking cessation.

Activity plans should be discussed, identifying the reasons for initial activity restriction and providing specific recommendations for progressive activity resumption during recovery. Return to work should be encouraged and planned for when appropriate (Pozen et al. 1977). Delineation of exercise programs and exercise facilities within the community and appropriate referral can help the patient implement the recommendations for physical activity. An important component of activity education is discussion of resumption of sexual intercourse, using as a general guideline that this is appropriate and safe at a time when other usual daily activities are reinstituted (Hellerstein and Friedman 1970; Stern et al. 1977). Patients are advised to use prophylactic nitroglycerin or nitrol ointment if sexual activity provokes angina; suggesting changes of position is inappropriate as little difference in cardiac work has been documented. Both partners should be counseled regarding resumption of sexual activity.

Patients should be taught about each medication they are to take once they return home — its name, purpose, dosage, the desired effects, and the potential untoward effects that require reporting to the physician. Many patients have not taken medication regularly prior to myocardial infarction, and the problems of medication-taking may be unfamiliar to them. Many other patients may be discharged home on a large number of fairly complex medication regimens; while the medication schedule should be simplified as much as feasible, the importance of taking medications regularly requires re-emphasis. Patients should also be taught the appropriate response to new or recurrent cardiac symptoms, emphasizing that immediate medical care is requisite for increased or prolonged chest discomfort. It is hoped that this approach may decrease the pre-hospital deaths from recurrent myocardial infarction. In recent years, many hospital centers in the United States have taught cardiopulmonary resuscitation (CPR) to families of myocardial infarction survivors, and the response has been extremely favorable. Family and patient appear to be reassured by this approach.

Finally, community resources should be defined for the patient and family as appropriate; these include counseling services, home-care agencies, guidance services, vocational rehabilitation facilities, and post-coronary educational groups or clubs. Discussions prior to discharge should review problems commonly encountered once the patient returns home, such as frequent overprotection by the family and possible negative community and job-related attitudes toward myocardial infarction or post-coronary bypass surgery patients; solutions should be suggested. Family counseling should include information about lifestyle adjustments to be anticipated during convalescence, focusing on the family's need to avert inappropriately restricting and unnecessarily invaliding the convalescent coronary patient.

Travel is usually deferred for 2 or 3 months following myocardial infarction or coronary bypass surgery. For patients whose occupation involves travel or who plan a vacation, counseling involves the need to always have available a summary of the medical record, a recent electrocardiogram, and an adequate supply of medication. A leisurely pace of travel is advised; identification should be made of a physician and medical center at the destination; and attention directed to appropriate cabin pressurization for air travel (Altman 1978).

Major patient and family concerns after return home typically relate to their understanding of tests or procedures planned for the early weeks, specific instructions about activity levels and return to work, and particularly what they can anticipate will occur over the subsequent months and years. Discussions with the patient prior to discharge from the hospital should thus reiterate explanations of these features.

Implementation and Methods

At Grady Memorial Hospital and the Emory University School of Medicine in Atlanta, Georgia, an algorithm for the education of the patient and family after myocardial infarction (Wenger and Mount 1974) is incorporated in the patient's medical record. It delineates the information to be taught at each stage of the illness; allows identification of the person doing the teaching, with notation of that individual's assessment of the patient's comprehension and learning; and identification of needs of the patient for additional teaching when the patient appears to have not fully accepted or comprehended the information. This format helps ensure that all requisite information is presented without inadvertent omissions, but avoids unnecessary duplication in teaching, while allowing repetition and reinforcement where required. It must be appreciated that this education occurs in the midst of complex emotional situations and adjustments, so that learning may be limited; considerable subsequent repetition, amplification, and reinforcement is typically necessary. However, an in-hospital teaching format is the cornerstone for subsequent education in the ambulatory phase.

In an effective educational program, the pattern of information presentation must be flexible enough to address problems perceived as relevant and meaningful by a particular patient at a particular time. Therefore, specific patient concerns and problems necessitate that some supplementary teaching be done on an individual basis, but the presentation of more general information appears best suited to a class or group format. Group teaching is economical of professional time and enables the patient to interact and share experiences with a peer group confronting similar problems. Active participation as a group member, through discussion and questioning, reinforces learning; functioning as a group member in realistic problem-solving and being able to help others is supportive of the patient's self-esteem at a time when the crisis of illness threatens the patient's self-image. This may be particularly important for the type A patient. Patients tend to be less anxious and self-conscious in a group setting than in an individual educational encounter; the peer group serves to facilitate adaption to stress and to decrease frustration. Control of these latter problems enhances and reinforces learning.

Audiovisual techniques and materials used in teaching both facilitate learning and provide a varied educational presentation — tape cassettes, slide-tape series, videotapes, etc. Test questions are often repeated at subsequent ambulatory care visits to assure that the information has been retained and understood. Research in the use of audiovisual materials indicates that about half of what is seen and heard tends to be remembered. Locally prepared materials have the advantage of portraying familiar surroundings and personnel. Take-home materials such as books, pamphlets, and instruction sheets reinforce the information presented during the hospitalization. Written directions for specific regimens of care are valuable reference material for the patient upon return home and help minimize conflicts between the patient and family that derive from vague or ambigous recommendations and instructions. The patient self-test, included as part of an audiovisual or printed presentation, appears to reinforce learning; when such a test is administered, a trained professional must be available to respond to any question or concerns the patient may have.

An encouraging and supportive attitude of the staff is necessary in all teaching encounters to help patients maintain their self-esteem and self-image while reasonably realistic plans are made to resume or, when necessary, to alter the former lifestyle. The staff must convey their respect for the patient, their concern for the patient as an individual; and emphasize that, in teaching, they are conferring some responsibility for care on the patient.

Despite intensive in-hospital education, additional repetition is needed after the patient returns home. Informational needs not perceived during the hospitalization become blatantly apparent at home when the patient must make decisions and solve problems related to health care. Also, even if the patient has adequately assimilated the cognitive material about the plans for care, the recommended changes in habit and lifestyle must be reviewed, evaluated, and finally incorporated into the patient's own value system when and where appropriate. Only then can the desired behavior changes be effected (Argondizzo 1978). A patient's attitudes and beliefs about the personal importance of a recommended component of therapy are major factors influencing compliance. Health professionals can provide the background information and help the patient acquire skills necessary for lifestyle change and health maintenance; they can guide the patient in setting realistic goals; and can offer continuing encouragement and support for health-related behavior, as well as serving as role models for this aspect. Nevertheless, it is the patient who must effect the changes. Patients and their families must become partners with the health professionals in both the preventive and the therapeutic care of their illness.

Expectations of Educational Programs

Recent data increasingly confirm that patients who understand their disease and the rationale for the components of its management have an increased incentive and an improved ability to cooperate in recommendations for health care (Linde and Janz 1979; Levine et al. 1979). Patients must be aware of what is expected of them and their areas of decision-making require definition. An education and counseling program helps delineate the patient's responsibility and role in the care of the cardiac illness, particularly as it relates to responses to new or recurrent symptoms and adherence to prescribed therapy.

Since many components of care for the patient with angina pectoris, after myocardial infarction, or after coronary bypass surgery, involve a long-term change in lifestyle and habits, intensive serial educational efforts appear appropriate. The late Dr. John Knowles, in defining preventive efforts as "forsaking the bad habits which many people enjoy," emphasized that major advances in health care will be enabled only "by what the individual is willing to do for himself . . ." (Knowles 1977).

References

Altman LK (1978) When a damaged heart is part of the vacation luggage. New York Times April 23

Argondizzo NT (1978) Patient and family education. In: Wenger NK, Hellerstein HK (eds) Rehabilitation of the coronary patient. Wiley & Sons, New York, p 117

Goble A (1969) Folklore and disability in heart disease. Cardiovasc Dis 5, 4

Hackett TP, Cassem NH (1976) White-collar and blue-collar responses to heart attack. J Psychosom Res 20:85

Hellerstein HK, Friedman EH (1970) Sexual activity and the post-coronary patient. Arch Intern Med 125:987

Knowles J (1977) Responsibility for health. Science 198:1103

Levine DM, Green LW, Deeds SG, Chivalow J, Russell RP, Finlay J (1979) Health education for hypertensive patients. JAMA 241:1700

Linde BJ, Janz NM (1979) Effect of a teaching program on knowledge and compliance of cardiac patients. Nurs Res 28:282

Mulcahy R, Hickey N, Graham I, McKenzie G (1975) Factors influencing long-term prognosis in male surviving a first coronary attack. Br Heart J 37:158

Pozen MW, Stechmiller JA, Harris W, Smith S, Fried DD, Voigt GC (1977) A nurse rehabilitator's impact on patients with myocardial infarction. Med Care 15:830

Salonen JT (1980) Stopping smoking and long-term mortality after acute myocardial infarction. Br Heart J 43:463

Stern MJ, Pascale L, Ackerman A (1977) Life adjustment post myocardial infarction: Determining predictive variables. Arch Intern Med 137:1680

Wallace N, Wallace DC (1977) Group education after myocardial infarction: Is it effective? Med J Aust 2:245

Weed LL (1974) A touchstone for medical education. Harv Med Alumni Bull November-December: 13–18

Wenger NK, Mount F (1974) An educational algorithm for myocardial infarction. Cardiovascular Nurs 10:11

Wilhelmsson C, Vedin JA, Elmfeldt D, Tibbin G, Wilhelmsson L (1975) Smoking and myocardial infarction. Lancet I:415

Is There Sufficient Appreciation of Vocational Counseling?

M. Niederberger, G. Czerwenka-Wenkstetten, and A. Eder

Introductory Remarks

From the physical point of view, vocational counseling depends on a precise diagnostic evaluation of the severity of underlying coronary artery disease and its prognostic implications, the severity of left ventricular impairment and the level of functional aerobic capacity. Usually the diagnostic evaluation is sufficiently appreciated, but in most instances insufficient use is made of this information for individual counseling. A major difficulty is that relatively little is known about the amount of physical stress which different professional activities — in different societies — impose on the cardiovascular system. Investigations have been made to define the aerobic power necessary to perform certain tasks, but adequate counseling would require actual measurements of heart rate and blood pressure in the individual patient during a number of different activities. We can propose that the peak heart rate during any physical activity should not exceed 85% of the maximal heart rate that has been determined individually during a symptom-limited maximal exercise test, whether performed on a bicycle ergometer or a treadmill. For longer periods, the heart rates should not exceed 75% of the individual maximal heart rate, and the average heart rate during a work day of 8 h should not exceed the heart rate that was reached by the individual at about 40% of his maximal working capacity.

While it is important to define the individual physical limits that should not be exceeded by the patient, it is also essential to give him the feeling of security and to acquaint him with the nature of coronary disease and the importance of symptoms such as angina and dyspnea. In a rehabilitation program the patient learns to interpret such symptoms so that he will be able to cope with them as soon as he experiences them during professional work. Therefore not only restraining the patient from physical stress, but also encouraging him to use his physical capacities properly is based on detailed diagnostic evaluation.

These statements, however, cover only a small portion of the overall problem. Our work has shown us that attempts to encourage patients to reorganize their lives in less stressful ways, for example by choice of new professional activities, were often bound to fail — even in cases where the new professional activities had been tested as to their requirements of heart rate and blood pressure.

What is it, then, that causes patients to neglect medical advice? A closer investigation of the psychosocial determinants that have led to the choice of a stressful professional situation in our patients' biographies concluded with two basic questions which must be answered for each patient:

a) Is there a tendency in patients that causes them to *cope with their reality* in a stressful way (i.e., in a way which gives them the impression of danger, which we may call distress)?

b) Are there processes that cause these individuals to *choose a stressful way of life*, for example by a choice of specific professional activities?

In other words, the two questions ca be put as follows:

a) Is "distress" in life something that depends more on the coping strategies of individuals than on objective factors "outside" the person, like physical requirements of the professional situation?

b) Is "distress" something that is being provoked systematically by patients because it serves a necessary function in their emotional lives?

Only in cases where both questions call for a negative answer can vocational counseling that gives patients an opportunity to change their "outer" world be a *direct* way to a solution of the psychosocial dilemma after the disease. Should we come to the conclusion that a patient either tends to interpret each possible world around him as stressful, or provokes "distress" in every possible world around him, a mere change of the *professional* situation cannot be expected to alter the patient's pathogenetic situation in any efficient way.

Theoretical Concepts: The Psychosocial Situation of Coronary Patients

A review of recent literature on the psychosocial situation co-determining the situation of coronary patients quite clearly reveals a picture of patients in whose lives stress plays a substantial role for their system of self-esteem and identity (Van der Valk 1967; Bastiaans 1968; Karstens 1970, cited by Uexküll et al. 1979). Psychoanalytic literature describes a number of typical psychosocial situations in patients with coronary heart diseases, such as: a discrepancy between actual ego and ego-ideal that causes substantial inner tensions (Korz-Rühling 1980). Other cases very clearly reveal the fact that patients tend to interpret any situation as stressful and deceptive and compensate these deceptions by a higher level of activity. Even a wife's tendency to stay asleep in the morning instead of making coffee was reported as a stressful event by one patient: it reactivated deceptive experiences of early childhood in the patient and led him to an interpretation of his world as cold and rejecting (Korz-Rühling 1980).

Therefore, the inability of coronary patients to be passive and dependent, which can be shown by the fact that most of them tend to overemphasize the importance of their professional work and even give up vacations, is based in their own tendency to interpret their world in a pathogenetic way (Korz-Rühling 1980).

Another aspect that is common for a number of coronary patients is their extended desire for control, which often finds an expression in the kind of profession that they are choosing. We learn from many cases that control over instruments and technical devices very often seems to have a substitutive function for affection and love (Goldschmidt 1980).

The high tendency to interpret their world in an abstract and intellectual manner very often leads them to a certain clumsiness in their personal relations. We often hear from these patients that they interpret their own personal relations to partners in a very difficult and complicated way: they over-intellectualize their emotions and thereby encounter a higher amount of double-binds and ambiguous situations in their emotional lives than other persons do (Goldschmidt 1980).

All these experiences give us strong evidence that stress and distress serve an integrative function in the personality system of coronary patients. We therefore must not be surprised when these patients react with great anxiety to attempts to change their life-style: in as much as they perceive stress as a touch stone for their efficiency, performance, and potency, taking away or reducing their stress implies a threat to their self-esteem.

Material and Methods

Coronary patients and persons of a control group (Table 1) were rated in their motivation for performance and activity, their feeling of being loved and emotionally accepted, their tendency to make excessive demands of their partners and family, their interpretation of their partner's behavior and their habits of using time.

Results

The ratings reveal a relatively clear picture (Table 2). Motivation for performance is high in 94% of the coronary patients, but only in 33% of the control group. Only 35% of the coronary patients feel emotionally accepted and loved, whereas 88% of the control group do. Ratings of the partner's reactions to the patient's behavior show that 88% of the coronary patients require a higher level of performance from their partners in professional work and in the home than the partners are motivated to.

Discussion

The results are highly significant. The items on which they are based have been selected from a large number of items in a pretest by the criterion of differentiating best the two groups of subjects according to our hypotheses. In this sense, our groups were "learning groups" and the results will have to be validated further in an independent material. However, we must be aware that such extremely high significances could in part be due to effects of the interviewing situation, which was characterized by a highly relaxed and confidential atmosphere due to the interviewers' (social assistants') attitudes and motivation.

Nevertheless, we see quite clearly from these data that in heart disease patients, emotionality is very often substituted by ideas of performance and control. Encouraging such persons simply to abstain from performance would obviously run counter to their motivational structure. Since we have no indication that the desire for emotionality is not present in these

Table 1. Subjects

	N Total	Age (yrs., mean value)	N Female	N Male	Diagnosis
Patients	51	52	18	33	Healed myocardical infarct (Average time elapsed after MI: 2.3 yrs.)
Controls	43	54	21	22	Healthy

Patients and controls did not differ significantly by age and sex distribution (T-Test)

Table 2. Results

	(1) Motivation for performance		(2) Feeling of acceptance emotionality		(3) Tendency to overcharge partners		(4) Constant time pressure		(5) Control over time		(6) Partner	
	High	Low	High	Low	High	Low	High	Low	Extern.	Intern.	"Zero"-p.	"Compet."
Coronary patients N (100%) = 51	94	6	35	65	88	12	100	0	92	8	51	49
Control group N (100%) = 43	33	67	88	12	49	51	56	44	26	74	23	77
Phi-coeff (measure of correlation)	0.65		- 0.54		0.50		0.55		0.68		0.20	

All correlations are significant at the 1% level ($p < 0.01$)

patients, we assume a typical way of skipping from affection to performance: Performance is offered by the patient, affection from others is expected as reward. In most of our cases, partners react with anxiety and fear of failure, since they interpret the patient's performance as a challenge to perform as highly as the patient does. Since the high level of performance of the patient mostly cannot be reached by partners, they react with anxiety and fear that keeps them from showing the desired affection. The patient feels that the reward was not as high as he expected, and feels an obligation to increase his own performance in order to elicit the expected result. By such a mutual misinterpretation of reactions the patient gets involved in a positive feedback loop of performance and fear that drives him to higher and higher performance.

Experiences of professional counselors yield a typical pattern of reaction of coronary patients to the heart attack: After a first period of panic, regression, fear and flight from any kind of activity whatsoever, which usually lasts 4–6 weeks, in a second period these patients tend to adopt the other extreme and go back to their former exaggerated level of activity, or in some instances even overcompensate and try to be more active than they were before. This reaction can easily be understood when we take into account that, according to some authors, the "narcistic offense" to these patients by the heart attack is extremely severe.

For vocational counseling therefore the crucial moment is when these patients decide to switch from complete passivity to hyperactivity; a moment which is usually very short and comes without warning. At this point, extended therapeutically oriented counseling is necessary. Before that point, the patient's resistance is usually too high, since he is still caught by the impression of danger for his life and narcistic disturbance. After that time, there is a risk that the counseling will be too late, since the already mentioned feedback of fear and performance has started to work again, and the patient's awareness is very often taken away by this process.

This model is quite compatible with the views of Köhle and Gauss (1979) who state that the anxiety of coronary patients is very often not so much a fear of death, but has its source in a threat to the regulative system of self-esteem (compare also Huebschmann 1966, 1967; Hackett 1968, cited by Uexküll 1979). The disease and its consequences are interpreted as a basic narcistic disturbance. Simultaneously, the loss of social esteem is feared. Patients for whose personality social esteem is a basic requirement see themselves deprived of the possibility of performing as highly as they deem necessary to get that esteem.

It is therefore necessary to point out that the same psychological factors which (according to Köhle and Gauss 1977 and other authors) lead to a higher risk of heart attack, also lead to the fact that the noxious consequences of the attack on the system of self-esteem are more severe in these patients. In other works, coronary patients have not only a higher risk of running into pathogenetic stress, they are also more exposed to threats to their self-esteem after the attack, whereby the dilemma after the attack is based on the same psychosocial factors that have helped to provoke the attack.

Conclusions

The main conclusion of these considerations and findings is clearly this: vocational counseling that tends to take away the patients' possibility of providing their social value through high performance, without giving them an opportunity to gain insight into their own strategies of coping and reinterpreting their social world, are bound to fail. Only if and when vocational counseling is an opportunity to show the patient that social status, affection and self-esteem can be gained through processes that are unrelated to performance, can coronary patients be expected to be ready to abstain from pathogenetic stress without fear of cracking their self-esteem.

Acknowledgement. G. Czerwenka-Wenkstetten was supported by a research grant from the *Bundesministerium für Wissenschaft und Forschung,* Vienna.

References

Bastiaans J (1968) Psychoanalytic investigations on the psychic aspects of acute myocardial infarction. Psychother Psychosom 16

Egger J (1980) Sexuelle Rehabilitation nach therapeutischer Neurologie und Psychiatrie für die Praxis. Perimed 5

Goldschmidt O (1980) Überlegungen zur Frage der Behandelbarkeit der Herzinfarktpatienten. In: Moersch et al. (ed)

Hackett TP (1977) Myocardinfakt: Emotionale Faktoren, die die Prognose verschlechtern (Interview). Tempo Med 1

Huebschmann H (1966) Vom Leiden organisch Herzkranker. Landarzt 42

Huebschmann H (1967) Zur psychopathologie von Patienten mit Herzinfarkt. Landarzt 43

Kartens R, Köhle K, Ohlmeier D, Weidlich S (1970) A multidisciplinary approach for the assessment of psychodynamic factors in young adults with acute myocardial infarctions. Psychother Psychosom 18

Krz-Rühling I (1980) Psychischer Konflikt. In: Moersch et al. (ed)

Köhle K, Gauss E (1979) Psychotherapie von Herzinfarktpatienten während der stationären und poststationären Behandlungsphase. In: Uexküll T (ed)

Moersch E, et al. (1980) Zur Psychopathologie von Herzinfarktpatienten. Psyche 6

Ringel E (1978) Selbstschädigung durch Neurose. Herder, Wien

Uexküll T et al. (1979) Lehrbuch der psychosomatischen Medizin. München Wien Baltimore

Van der Valk JM, Groen IJ (1967) Personality structure and conflict situation in patients with myocardial infarctions. J Psychosom Res 11

Can We Improve the Prognosis of Coronary Heart Disease?

J.J. Kellermann

General Considerations

Atherosclerosis starts at an early age and while the atherosclerotic process has been shown to be reversible in vitro and in animal studies, the final evidence of the reversibility in humans is still lacking and the data on the regression in humans are difficult to interpret. The pathogenesis of atherosclerosis as the cause of coronary artery disease is still uncertain. Those who believe that the reversal of hyperlipidemic conditions may cause a regression of the atherosclerotic state, must consider the fact that atherosclerosis in humans may be due to a multiplicity of causes and not just to hypercholesterolemia, as in the experimental atherosclerosis induced in animals.

Furthermore, we should remember that genetic factors contribute to the pathogenesis of coronary atherosclerosis. This has been confirmed in prevalence studies among genetically different groups, living under similar environmental conditions, as well as in the high incidence of coronary artery disease in first degree relatives, especially if the parents were diseased when young.

A high concordance for myocardial infarction in identical twins (44% for monozygotic twins and 14% for dizygotic twins) has been observed. Finally, a close association has been found with one or more genetically determined risk factors, such as hypercholesterolemia, diabetes mellitus, hypertension, personality traits, and others.

Epidemiologic Considerations

Of late, we have been confronted with a systematic decrease in mortality due to coronary artery disease between 1968 and 1977, especially in the U.S., Finland, New Zealand, Norway, Canada, Israel, and some other countries.

The investigators who believe that there is ample evidence that the decrease in mortality in the above countries may be due to an effectice control of risk factors, i.e., decrease in cigarette smoking, control of hypertension and diabetes, change in food intake and intensive physical training, must take into consideration the fact that similar efforts in risk factor modifications were made in other countries too, such as Poland, Yugoslavia, Ireland, Denmark, France, and others. In these latter countries a systematic increase in mortality from coronary artery disease has been observed in the same time period.

The question then arises of whether it is possible that the epidemic of coronary heart disease is declining. In this respect we should like to quote Ivan Illich in his "Limits of Medicine" in which he stated that "the study of evolution of diseased patterns provides evidence that, during the last century, doctors have affected epidemics no more profoundly than priests during early times. Epidemics came and went, imprecated by both, but touched by neither."

Mortality figures are still not reliable when discussing a possible decrease of a disease pattern, without taking into consideration morbidity rates. Unfortunately, such rates are yet not available and therefore it is rather questionable at this stage whether indeed the decreased mortality is caused by the general trend of the decreased number of persons with coronary artery disease, or a more efficient conservative and surgical therapy, as well as a proper management of the coronary patient in the acute stage.

Primary Prevention

When considering a possible alteration of prognosis of coronary heart disease, the effect of multifactorial primary prevention programs should be discussed. We are aware of the great number of risk factors and their possible influence on morbidity of coronary heart disease. In the past few years Morris and Pfaffenbarger found that vigorous high intensity activity may have a protective rather than a selective influence on reinfarction rates. Others have shown that vigorous exercise, such as long distance running, and high intensity training, increases HDL cholesterol. Furthermore, there may be a great number of biases involved in all kinds of primary prevention programs, while it is probable that the control of smoking, hypertension, and hypercholesterolemia may eventually influence the natural course of the disease. No scientific evidence can be offered as to the dominant or primary factor responsible for the clinical outburst of coronary heart disease or of sudden death. It seems that there are still a number of unknown risk factors which may prove as important as the known ones. In considering the very important studies of Morris and Pfaffenbarger, one should analyse the composition of the population involved in such studies. It is obvious that the individual who is able to maintain a routine vigorous physical training for many years will differ from the viewpoint of health hygiene motivation, discipline, and probably also a general philosophy of life from others who believe that you can be lazy and still remain healthy and fit. In order to illustrate this remark we should like to mention a kibbutz study undertaken by us 10 years ago and involving 2952 individuals. We have found that only 17 individuals fulfilled the criterions of vigorous physical activity performed at leisure time. Out of the total population examined, 80% were of European origin, 15% were Israeli born, while the remaining 5% were of Asian origin. Of the 17 individuals involved extensively in sport activities, ten, or about 60%, were of Asian origin, an ethnic group having in general a lower incidence of coronary heart disease. In further consideration of Pfaffenbarger's longshoremen study, we should like to add that almost all of the individuals involved in vigorous activity were agricultural workers. In this small group, which is probably a nonrepresentative sample, all had initially normal blood pressure, were nonsmokers, and had rather low serum cholesterol levels. In a 5-year follow-up none of them developed clinical C.H.D. Knowing that we are talking only about a very small group, we would like to point out that one should analyze in detail the composition of the population under study, in order to avoid justified criticism of preselected intervention groups.

In discussing the possibility of the influence of primary prevention on morbidity and longevity, one should mention that there probably exist a number of factors which remain unknown and that intervention must start in childhood by changing basic educational concepts and teaching the principles of health hygiene and applying the excellent advice of ancient doctors regarding the preservation of health.

A B C Typology

Increasing interest arose with regard to the influence of the psychosocial stresses and personality traits on the incidence of C.H.D. While the so-called type A personality has more than double higher incidence of C.H.D. when compared to type B, in a number of countries these findings have not been confirmed. In a study performed by our group, we found that a number of kibbutz managers showed a greater coronary risk under relatively tranquil nonstressful conditions. They appeared to thrive from the point of view of their risk factor profiles when under greater stress. We therefore thought that we have demonstrated a type C personality, that is, a coronary prone person in the absence of the kinds of conditions a type A person is likely to seek out for themselves. The question may be posed regarding whether or not it is feasible that ethnic, social, and cultural structures influences behavior patterns can be altered from childhood with an ultimate goal decreasing C.H.D. incidence.

Secondary Prevention

The third question deals with the effect of a comprehensive intervention program in coronary patients.

It is well established that it is possible to improve cardiocirculatory performance and psychological conditions in patients with signs and symptoms of C.H.D. The prognosis of these patients is, in the first line dependent on the appearance of various clinical events, such as myocardial infarction, angina pectoris, and congestive heart failure, in addition to the presence of major risk and genetic factors. While there is a lack of scientific evidence regarding whether or not comprehensive rehabilitation programs have a beneficial influence on morbidity and longevity, a randomized study in Finland (Kallio et al.), as well as two of our own controlled but nonrandomized studies, have shown that there is a decrease in mortality in the intervention group. It must, of course, be stated that we are talking about preselected members of the population less than 65 years old. In order to avoid justified criticism, we have lately implemented another study involving 330 patients with angina pectoris in the age range of 27 to 65 years. The patients were divided into two major groups, according to *their angina pectoris threshold heart rate* (A.T.H.R.). Group A consisted of patients with an A.T.H.R. of 120 b/min and above, and group B of patients with A.T.H.R. less than 120 b/min (see Table 1).

A 5-year-follow up was undertaken. This included a control group which visited our outpatients clinic once or twice per year and received conventional drug therapy such as nitrites, beta blockers, and calcium antagonists, and an intervention group undergoing a continuous comprehensive rehabilitation program. This program includes risk factor modification, cessation of smoking, weight control, physical training, drug therapy, and systematic clinical

Table 1. Five-year follow-up in patients with angina pectoris (N = 283)

	Outpatients without rehabilitation N = 159	Continuously supervised rehabilitation N = 124
Unchanged	44.6	64.5
Reinfarction	11.3	7.2
Surgery	12.6	11.5
Died	17.6	4.8

observations and reassessment. The patients in this groups visited our institute at least twice per week.

A third group included patients who underwent only a 16-week rehabilitation program and were then discharged from the program, but followed up for another 5 years.

The following mortality rates found were:

In the group A.T.H.R. 120 and above:

  8.3%   for the control group,

13.8%   for the short-time rehabilitation group

  2.5%   for the continuous rehabilitation group.

In the group of patients who developed pain at a heart rate of less than 120:

25.3%   in the control group

27.3%   in the short-time rehabilitation group

  9.3%   in the continuous rehabilitation group.

In a recently completed study consisting of 229 patients after transmural myocardial infarction, who underwent a long-term multifactorial intervention program (mean age at admission 49 ± 4 years), a very low mortality rate was found. The follow-up lasted 5.6 ± 3.5 years. It should be mentioned that total cholesterol, and systolic and diastolic blood pressure decreased significantly during follow-up. Of previous smokers (77.4%) 66.5% stopped the habit. Of the total 229 patients, 46 interrupted the program during follow-up. Of the latter number, 38 discontinued the program for nonmedical reasons, such as moving to another locality, lack of motivation, or a busy professional schedule. Of these nonmedical dropouts, two patients died in the follow-up period (mean age at death, 65.5 years). Eight patients discontinued the program because of clinical deterioration such as increasing angina, cardiac failure, or reinfarction. Six of these eight patients died, a mean of 3.3 ± 2.0 years after discontinuing the program (mean age at death, 59 ± 3.2 years). The intervention group (the remaining 183 patients) had a mortality rate of 3.2% within the follow-up period (0.6% each year; mean age at death, 51.1 ± 5 years) (see Table 2).

This is a preliminary communication; further analysis of the results is needed, but, as in our previous reports, mortality is very low. It can be argued that the high-rsik patients had been taken out of the study after 4.1 years of intervention. Nonetheless, if we include all patients who died from a cardiac cause (both members of the intervention group and dropouts), the mortality is still significantly lower (1.3% each year) than the mortality rates of our non-randomized control groups (2.4% and 2.7% each year, respectively). It seems to us that the multifactorial approach may be, in part, responsible for the low mortality rates in this recent study. To exclude the great number of biases interfering with analysis seems almost impossible.

Table 2. Continuous rehabilitation program

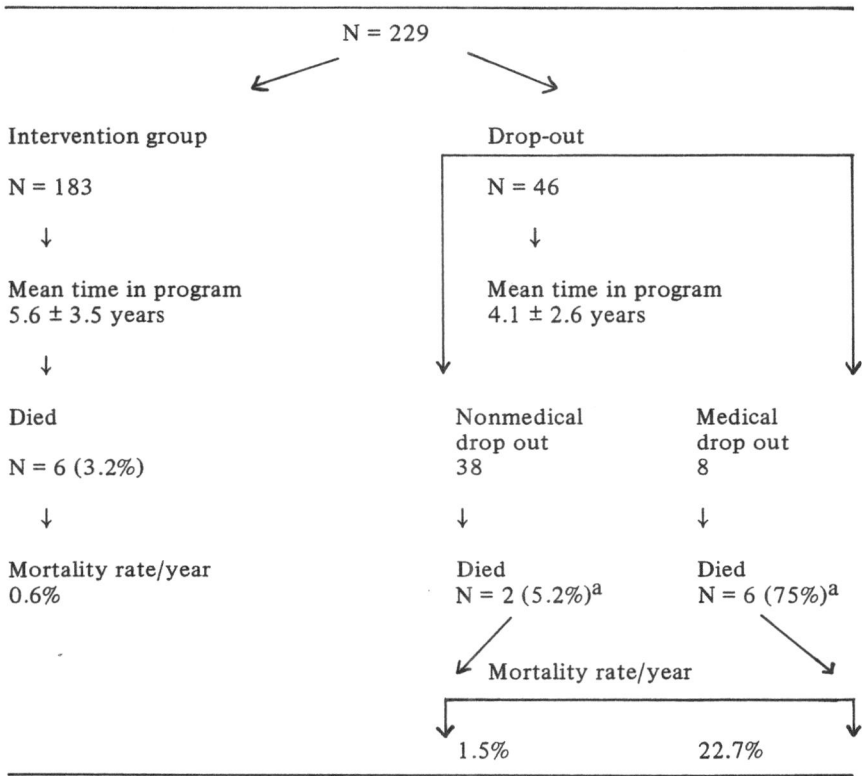

a   Mean time lapse after discontinuation of program. 3.3 ± 2.0 years

These results would indicate that mortality may be influenced by comprehensive intervention programs in selected patients with overt CHD. We still do not know whether or not it is possible to influence the dynamic course of the disease. When and why are we facing a clinical outburst or a rapid deterioration of the disease?

Is it sudden emotional stress, extreme physical strain, uncontrollable environmental change, or sudden unbalanced conditions involving the autonomic nervous system and or the intercellular metabolism.

In conclusion we would like to state the following: May it be that we have reached a peak in this epidemic of modern times and that from now on the plague is on the decrease, as indicated by reduced mortality in a number of countries. May it be that the improves management of the coronary patients in the acute phase, and the comprehensive coronary care utilized in many countries, resulted in the retreat of mortality rates. There are still a great number of questions to be asked and more hard facts and less theories are needed before we can answer – if at all – the provocative question of whether or not prognosis of coronary artery disease can be altered.

Summary

In analyzing a possible alteration of prognosis in CHD, one has to consider: (a) whether it can be demonstrated that an atherosclerotic process in the human is reversible; (b) whether modification of risk factors and change in habits can influence the natural course of the disease; and (c) whether any therapeutic modality such as drugs, exercise, or surgery have any influence on morbidity and longevity. As *to the first question:* The notion that atherosclerosis is a reversible process was suggested 60 years ago. While in animal studies atherosclerotic processes have been reversed, the data available to date about a regression in the human are rather incomplete and there still exist considerable problems regarding interpretation. As to *the second question,* on the effect of the modification of risk factors, it can be agreed that hyperlipidemia, hypertension, and smoking are major risk factors in relation to the incidence of CHD. Epidemiologic studies have shown that individuals without these major risks had a significantly lower CHD incidence. Based on these assumptions, major intervention studies have been implemented in various parts of the world, with the aim of combating smoking habits, controlling food intake, and efficiently treating hypertension. In some countries a systemic decrease in CHD mortality in the past 5 years has been observed. Despite the still high incidence, it seems obvious that mortality of CHD is declining. Answers to the question of whether or not risk factor modification and change in life style, or a more effective therapy are responsible for this decline, seem to be ambiguous. One can try to imply a deductive method of analysis and assume that risk factor control may influence the prognosis in some individuals, and slow down the dynamics of the natural course of the disease. The reply to *the third question* allows a great deal of speculation. Comprehensive secondary prevention programs, as applied in many centers of the world, have shown that, for example, exercise therapy can reduce or prevent the clinical manifestation of the disease (A.P. and/or reinfarction), by other mechanisms than a direct effect on coronary atherosclerotic processes. Exercise therapy has been shown to have beneficial influences on hemodynamic parameters, cardiocirculatory performance, and risk factor modification, to increase emotional stability, and to reduce anxiety. Comprehensive rehabilitation based on long-term intervention and follow-up has, in some studies, resulted in a lower mortality. Beta blockers have been shown to reduce infarct size when applied at an early stage. Ectopic rhythm has been suppressed, especially in individuals with frequency-induced ectopy, and therefore there may be a possible influence in preventing sudden death. It was repeatedly stated that coronary surgery, as a rehabilitative measure, may have a beneficial influence on quality of life. There is little doubt that aortocoronary bypass operations applied in main vessel and progressive three-vessel disease, have an influence on longevity as well. In these latter patients, prognosis can be altered unquestionably. A number of theories and working hypotheses are available to date, but only a few facts, therefore it would seem bold to formulate a plain reply to the posed question.

References

1   Hayet M, Kellerman JJ (1981) The angina pectoris threshold heart rate as a prognostic sign. Results of five years follow-up. Cardiology 2
2   Illich I (1977) Limits to medicine. Pelican Books, London, p 23
3   Kellermann JJ (1975) Rehabilitation of patients with coronary heart disease. Prog Cardiovasc Dis 17:303—328

4   Kellermann JJ, Denolin H (1977) Critical evaluation of cardiac rehabilitation. Karger, Basel
5   Kellermann JJ (1978) Modulated sympathetic stimulation as a feature within the framework of comprehensive rehabilitation in patients with coronary heart disease. In: Gross F (ed) Modulation of sympathetic tone in the treatment of cardiovascular disease. Huber, Bern, pp 293–299
6   Levy RE, Fenleib M (1980) Risk factor for coronary artery disease and their management. In: Braunwald E (ed) Heart disease. Saunders, Philadelphia, pp 1246–1278
7   Morris JN, Chave SPW, Adam C, Sirey C (1973) Vigorous exercise in leisure time and the incidence of coronary heart disease. Lancet 1:333–338
8   Pfaffenbarger RS, Brand RJ, Sholtz RI, Jung DL (1978) Energy expenditure, cigarette smoking and blood pressure level as related to death from specific disease. Am J Epidemiol 108:12–18
9   Wintner I, Kellermann JJ (1976) Psychological factors involved in cardiac rehabilitation. In: Stocksmeier U (ed) Psychological approach to the rehabilitation of coronary patients. Springer, Berlin Heidelberg New York, pp 156–172
10 Eden D, Shirom A, Kellermann JJ, Aronson J, French JRP (1976) Stress, anxiety and coronary risk in a supportive society. In: Spielberger, Sarson (eds) Stress and anxiety. Hemisphere, Washington D C, pp 251–268

Institutionalized, Residential Rehabilitation of Patients with Ischemic Heart Disease?

M.J. Halhuber and K. König

In this paper I shall deal with my subject in four main sections:
1. Endpoints (What are the goals?)
2. Methods of cardiac rehabilitation (How?)
3. Some results of institutional rehabilitation (Hoehenried long-term study).
4. Conclusions and consequences.

Three Endpoints of Cardiac Rehabiliation (what are its aims?)

Medical Physiologic Aims

Rehabiliation is intended to compensate irreparable consequences by still present functions of the organism. This statement refers not only to the cardiac and extracardiac possibilities of compensation of cardiac damage, but also to the interactions of loss and compensation within the somatic or psychosocial scope. The phenomenon of functional compensation is of central importance in rehabilitation.

Social-Psychological Aims

The original meaning of rehabilitation is "restoring of honor." In our society this means the restoration of ones "Honor of achievement", ones social status, ones role within the society. Rehabilitation compromises all somatic and psychosocial endeavors to preserve for the person afflicted with a chronic heart disease, the same position within society that he occupied before his afflication. Problems of keeping the job, of protection against being discharged, of being reemployed, the modification of the work load, or relocation — rarely — of retraining, and finally, of being retired and how to cope with it, are of the greatest importance for those endeavors.

Epidemiologic Aims

Secondary (and tertiary) prevention: to decelerate the process of heart disease and to prevent complications.

Methods of Cardiac Rehabilitation (how do we achieve these aims?)

Do cardiologists agree about the need for a rehabilitation program which satisfies the recommendations of the WHO and the International Society of Cardiology ("as early, as long, as comprehensive as possible")? Probably they disagree about the way in which it is organized. We distinguish four types of care after a patient's discharge from the general hospital:

Informal Approach

The patient is advised by his/her doctor but there is no supervised program. R. Mulcahy defines this as ". . . a personal and individualized approach without the use of formal laboratory or other procedures. For example, no routine exercise testing or formal group classes are employed. Emphasis is on 'normal' or physiologic exercise such as walking, cycling and golf". This informal approach differs from the following method by the fact that it is based on advising (Mulcahy 1981).

Supervised Out-Patient Coronary Group Therapy

Group therapy can be carried out through being a member of the coronary club or by participation in a supervised exercise program (Wenger and Hellerstein 1978, Halhuber C. 1980).

Institutional Early Rehabilitation in a Specialized Center

With regard to this subject, see Halhuber M. (1969).

Supervised Group Therapy Following Institutionalized Residential Rehabilitation in a Specialized Center or a Rehabilitation Unit of a General Hospital

We think we should distinguish these four different approaches to rehabilitation after myocardial infarction to avoid misunderstandings in the discussion between antagonists and protangonists, but there is less controversy in reality than is apparent from a theoretical standpoint. A supervised out-patient coronary group with three sessions (of 2 h) a week is close to our concept of an early residential rehabilitation in a specialized center.

Arguments in Favor of Residential Rehabilitation

Diagnostic Arguments. The following diagnostic procedures are more easily achieved in a specialized center or unit than in the hospital or by the family doctor:
1. Stress testing and ergometry or telemetry under controlled "daily life" conditions. (At the center of Hoehenried 90 000 bicycle ergometry tests have been done without fatal accidents).
2. Long-term Holter-monitoring (24 h) to identify dangerous arrhythmias during controlled "daily life activities".
3. Micro catherization (floating Swan-Ganz catheter) during exercise to identify an early heart failure, should suspicious symptoms or signs occur during daily activities.

4. Integration of coronary angiography and other invasive procedures in the diagnostic program at the most suitable period for evaluation.

Health Education. "We probably have to achieve maximal risk factor reduction to be effective in CDH patients after infarction. We probably have to achieve multiple risk factor reduction to have any significant impact on the rate of reinfarction" (Blackburn 1978). The patient has to learn (information) and to accept (motivation) a new personal behavior pattern (life style) concerning not only indivial risk factors but also daily medication. It is well known that only 58% of all patients after myocardial infarction regularly take their pills. Self-motivation, for example, discipline during the individual build-up of a long-term drug regimen, is supported by mutual motivation of the group. This is especially important for smokers and obese people.

Psychology and Social Therapy. Many problems concerning anxiety, depression, denial, and overmotivation have to be mastered after a heart attack (Hackett 1978). Daily group therapy sessions, individual counseling by the doctor and even by the primary therapists (nurse, etc.) are as helpful as are daily sessions of progressive muscle relaxation. In our experience the patient learns more easily in new surroundings than at home to adjust to a new life style in his private life (family counseling, dietary advice, sex counseling, leisure time planning) and professional life (vocational counseling, selective placement, and job planning). For this purpose specialized social workers and psychologists are involved.

Exercise Therapy Arguments. Starting daily exercise therapy after discharge from the general hospital often makes the patient feel anxious, depressed, and insecure. We believe that physiotherapy is also a special type of psychotherapy. In a supervised rehabilitation program the patient learns to know his possibilities and limits, to gain self-confidence, to lose his anxiety, and to avoid dangerous over-motivation.

The following figures demonstrate some results regarding the physiologic effects of exercise therapy. These results involve a 4–6 week rehabilitation period in 1200 patients from the rehabilitation center in Waldkirch/West Germany (König, 1977). As it is well-known, a good measure of the improvement in the work that the heart does is represented by the product of blood pressure and pulse. The patients were subdivided into groups. In group A, infarction had occurred less than 3 months previously. In group B, it had occurred between 3 and 12 months before entering the group, and in group C the time between infarction and rehabilitation was more than 12 months. The latter cases involved repeated treatment in the rehabilitation center. The decrease in the blood pressure-pulse product during the period of training at a submaximal load was still significant in all three groups. The figure was the highest in group A at 10.8% and came down to 9% in group C. The improvement in the heart's working economy by means of physical training has the expected effect of increasing fitness (Fig. 1).

At the end of the 4–6 week rehabilitation period, the maximal oxygen pulse increased in group A by 38%. This enormous increase in physical performance at the beginning of phase II is understandable since infarction had occurred only a relatively short time before. Therefore, the patients still showed a very reduced performance at the beginning of the training therapy. As expected, in the later stages of rehabilitation the rates of increase were only 14% and 10%. All increases in performance are statistically highly significant (Fig. 2).

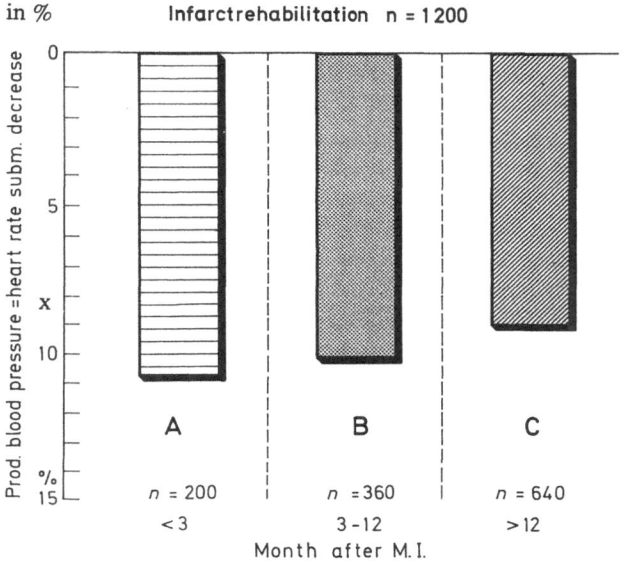

Fig. 1

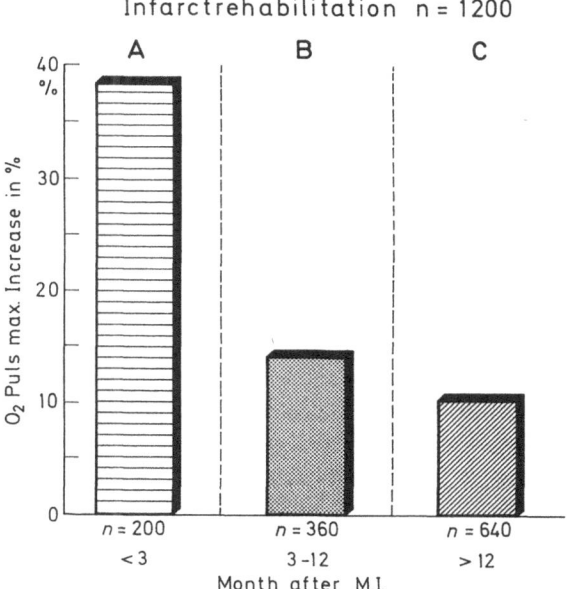

Fig. 2

A very interesting result was obtained by measuring the radiologically determined heart volume before and after the 4—6 week rehabilitation period (Fig. 3).

In all three groups there were highly significant reductions in heart size. Again the most pronounced reduction was found in the patients of group A at the beginning of phase II.

One argument explaining the statistically highly significant reduction in heart size is that in the acute infarction phase a compensatory enlargement of the heart occurs in the sense of Frank Starling mechanism depending on the size of the scar and hence on the loss of contractile substance. In this case the enlargement can be connected to a reduction in contractility and an increase in ventricular filling pressure. The reduction in size of the heart means that the loss of contraction of the scar has been compensated by the remaining healthy myocardium. The reduction in heart size is only in part the consequence of simultaneous digitalization. The analyses have shown that even without digitalis significant reductions in heart size were observed (K. König, unpublished).

Some Preliminary Results from a Long-term Study to Support this "Philosophy"

The Hoehenried myocardial infarction study started in 1970. Today it covers more than 1300 MI patients, who are reexamined every 6 months. The physicians performing the examinations do a complete medical evaluation and test the patients in their everyday life activities. Together with psychologists we tried to determine correlations among physical, psychological, and social date, following the WHO interdisciplinary definition of health. All patients were integrated in a comprehensive rehabilitation program: After discharge from the acute hospital the MI patient comes as soon as is feasible to the rehabilitation center. During the first 4—6 weeks he/she underwent physical training, and was adjusted to the appropriate medication. Group therapy was administered, and social workers assisted in solving any social problems. After leaving the rehabilitation center the patients were followed by two check-ups a year.

Mortality

An intermediate analysis made after 6 years of the intended 10-year study with 345 patients shows a yearly mortality rate of 2.12% (H. Angster, R. Glonner 1979). This mortality rate is comparable to the natural history of a one-vessel disease. The mortality rate of these postinfarct patients is less than twice the general mortality rate of the age-adjusted population in Germany. It is to be expected that more than half of all postinfarct patients suffer from a two- or three-vessel disease. Our 6-year survival rate seems therefore to indicate a positive effect of our rehabilitation system.

Comparable studies with similar diagnosis, of the same social class of patients, the same age and sex, but not undergoing the same type of rehabilitation techniques, showed a yearly mortality rate of about 4% (W. Oberwittler, H. Schulte 1975). It is difficult to compare different studies due to different processes of selection and there exist no real control groups. We believe that our favourable mortality rate and its undeniable differences to that obtained in other studies, is attributed to more than just a propitious selection of our patients (H. Angster, R. Glonner 1979).

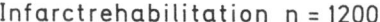

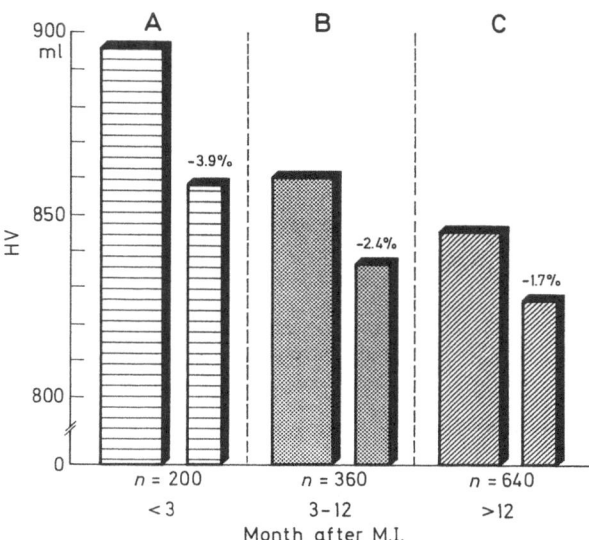

Fig. 3

Infarctrehabilitation n = 1200

Significance for all differences p < 0.001

Return to Work

The patients of the Hoehenried myocardial infarction study are not different from a comparable population in Bavaria as regards family, status, education, and number of children. This is important because we can at least give representative results for the postinfarct patients in Bavaria. We found that patients doing unskilled work change jobs more frequently, have more financial problems, and suffer from professional downgrading more than the others. Since we know that stresses resulting from this situation are important risk factors for a reinfarction, we should give these patients more attention (H. Angster, R. Glonner 1979) (Fig. 4).

Truck drivers get four times, hall porters three times, and salesmen (especially traveling salesmen) twice as many infarctions as expected by the contribution of these professions in the normal community. One of the common characteristics of truck drivers, hall porters, and salesmen is the lack of physical activity in these jobs (F. Hauss, U. Stocksmeier 1976).

Long-term studies in Germany without an institutionalized rehabilitation, report a rate of return to work which is only 50% as compared to more than 80% for blue collar workers and 90% for white collar workers in our study, using an institutionalized residential system with regular follow-up (Stabl, Stocksmeier, Natus 1980). From an epidemiologic point of view the group of Oberwittler is an adequate control group for our study with comparable age, social class, sex, and time of the study. The methodological difference is that Oberwittler and co-workers check the patients only to see what happened after several years whilst we intervened as often as necessary and rechecked patients twice a year. The big difference in the rate of return to work after MI (62%—86%) seems to support a compre-

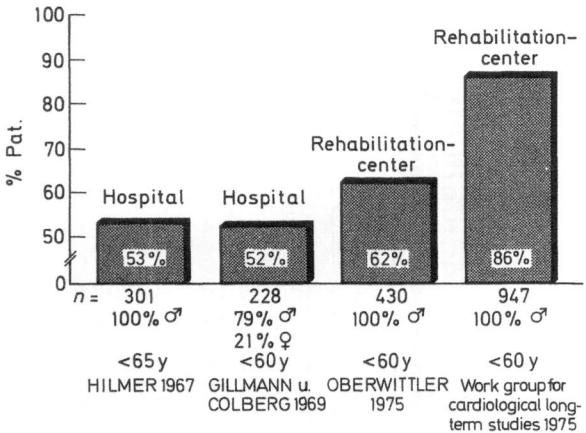

Fig. 4. Return to work after myocardial infarction. Data from various studies

hensive system of rehabilitation as described (W. Oberwittler, H. Schulte 1975). Not only is the percentage of patients returning to work important, but also the percentage of patients continuing their jobs: In our study more than 50% still continued their work after 5 years.

The different groups in our country report similar results: 60% of postinfarct patients return to work without institutionalized rehabilitation and 80% with a comprehensive program. F. Kubicek reports that among 800 patients in Vienna, Austria, 75.8% of white collar workers and 58% of blue collar workers returned to work following his comprehensive program (F. Kubicek 1976). We believe that there are more socio-economic than medical reasons for different results in different countries.

Change of Risk Factors and Quality of Life

It is our hypothesis that patients adjust more easily in new surroundings than at home, to a new style in their dietary habits, medication, physical activity, family relationships, and professional attitudes. During the comprehensive rehabilitation in the center, we can demonstrate a highly significant reduction of all known risk factors (blood pressure, smoking, cholesterol and triglycerides, and body weight) during their stay in the rehabilitation center phase, and that the out-patient follow-up was able to keep these values low over a period of 4 years (Fig. 5a–c), (Table 1) (Halhuber M, Stocksmeier U 1976).

We believe that in the future it will become a new, but very important, methodoligical principle to measure the quality of life after a heart attack. That means measuring not only the medical influence on psychological attitudes of the patient. (In our concept of cardiac rehabilitation the intention os to optimize personalization and socialization of cardiac patients). Therefore we have to measure by new psychological methods how anxiety, depression, denial, overmotivation, and coronary-prone behavior patterns are changing.

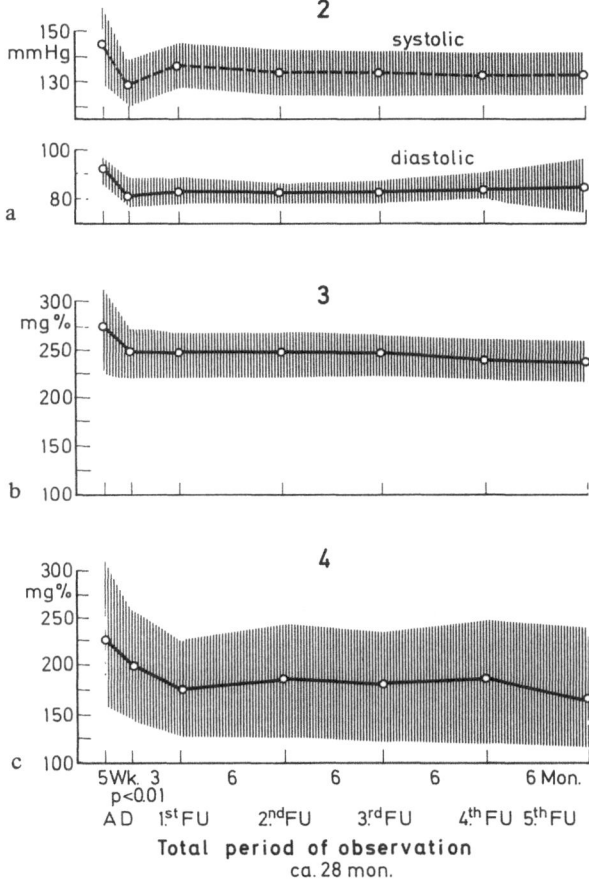

Fig. 5a–c. Development of risk factors in myocardial infarction patients of the Hoehenried Rehabilitation Center. **a** Systolic and diastolic blood pressure (n = 293); **b** levels of cholesterol (n = 293); **c** levels of triglycerides (n = 282). *A*, admission; *D*, discharge; *FU*, follow-up

Cost-Benefit Relationship

It is very difficult to compare the cost-benefit relationships between different medical systems. Therefore I would like to make only the following statement concerning the situation in West Germany with its developed social insurance system:

The cost-benefit relationship is more than favorable, if by the rehabilitation system a delay in the payment of the sick pension of 1 year is achieved.

Costs of 6 weeks in a rehabilitation center	DM 5 000.00
Pension for 1 year (white collar)	DM 12 000.00
to	DM 14 000.00
Pension for 1 year (blue collar)	DM 10 000.00
Gross domestic product for 1976 in West Germany	DM 45 000.00

Table 1. Risk factors present on admission (of inpatients) to Hoehenried Rehabilitation Center and the mean values of 8—10 6-monthly follow-up examinations

	On admission to the center (%)	Mean values of 8—10 follow-up examinations (%)
Hypertension	23.3	5.8
Overweight	79.5	67.0
(More than 10% overweight)	(50.0)	(34.9)
Cigarette smoking	69.5	25.3
Heavy smoking (15—30 cigarettes)	50.9	6.4
Hypercholesterolemia (over 280 mg%)	42.6	16.8
Hypertriglyceridemia	53.5	37.9
Hyperuricemia (8—12 mg%)	5.0	9.8

Conclusions

According to S.M. Fox III (1978) there are four levels of acceptance of regimes:
1. Proven: Beyond reasonable doubt
2. Prudent action: Justified by substantional, although incomplete data and acceptly low hazard
3. Promising: But more data needed
4. Possible: Hypothesis only

I think it is justified to range the actual possibilities of cardiac rehabilitation between 2 and 3, but closer to the level of "prudent action".

What practical consequences seem to be important?
1. Residential rehabilitation of MI patients in a specialized institution is a good, pleasant, effective, and efficient method to start a change of habit (smoking, diet, et.c).
2. In the future, every general hospital with a coronary care unit (CCU) will also need a rehabilitation care unit (RCU), or close cooperation with a specialized rehabilitation center. Such a specialized department will have diagnostic, therapeutic, and economic advantages for the patient who remains in the same organizational frame work), and for the training of young docturs in rehabilitation during his or her postgraduate educational program (the student remains in the same educational system).
3. Out-patient coronary group therapy and follow-up reevaluation seem to constitute a prolonged behavioral therapy. Regular reexaminations are positive reinforcements for the patient. This "open, but organized rehabilitation" seems to us the most effective way of reinforcing the results of the initial phase of residential rehabilitation in a specialized center or specialized unit of the acute hospital.
4. The most important point in the rehabilitation program is the quality and quantity of contact between patient and doctor. The involvement of a single devoted doctor in health education (information and motivation) can replace most of the advantages of an institution or organized group.

5. More research is needed with an interdisciplinary, and international multicenter approach to this problem. Antagonists and protagonists of the need for institutionalized residential establishments suffer from a lack of information concerning methodological problems, especially appropriate control groups, efficiency in changing risk factors and life habits, and finally cost effectiveness.

Summary

In this paper we tried to summarize our experience with 14 years of institutionalized cardiac rehabilitation in the rehabilitation center for diseases of the heart in Hoehenried near Munich. These experiences and the results of a long-term study of more than 1000 myocardial infarction patients support the hypothesis that after the patients' discharge from the general hospital, any out-patient coronary group therapy (anti-coronary club) should be preceded by an early residential rehabilitation in a specialized center which could be a unit of a general hospital. The prognosis, and especially the quality of life of a patient with coronary heart disease, seems to be improved by changing the risk factors and total life situation (including bypass surgery as a measure of rehabilitation). The task of improving the personal life style of the patient and of changing his/her habits (smoking, overeating, physical inactivity, emotional attitudes) needs the special conditions of group psychotherapy and health education. These conditions are more easily achieved in a specialized residential rehabilitation unit than in the traditional ward of a general hospital or in the usual out-patient clinics.

References

Angster H, Glonner R (1979) Medizinische und berufliche Rehabilitation Herzinfarkt durch umfassende Nachbetreuung. Landes-Versicherungsanstalt Oberbayern, München

Blackburn H (1978) In: Wenger NK, Hellerstein HK (eds) Rehabilitation of the coronary patient. John Wiley and Sons, New York Chichester Brisbane Toronto

Fox SM (1978) In: Wenger NK, Hellerstein HK (eds) Rehabilitation of the coronary patient. John Wiley and Sons, New York Chichester Brisbane Toronto

Hackett TP (1982) Coping with the problems of convalescence following myocardial infarction. In: Mathes P, Halhuber M (eds) Controversies in cardiac rehabilitation. Springer, Berlin Heidelberg New York

Halhuber C (1980) Rehabilitation in ambulanten Koronargruppen. Springer, Berlin Heidelberg New York

Halhuber M (1969) Für und Wider Anschlußheilmaßnahmen nach Herzinfarkt. Deutsche Rentenversicherung 1:1

Halhuber M, Stocksmeier U (1976) Herzinfarktrehabilitation. Internistische Praxis 16:829

Hauss F, Stocksmeier U (1976) Sozialdemographische Daten von Herzinfarktpatienten. Münchner Med Wochenschr 32:1007

König K (1977) Changes in physical capacity, heart size and function in patients after myocardial infarction, who underwent a 4–6 week physical training program. Cardiology 62:232

Kubicek F, Blazek G, Blum J, Gaul G (1976) Ambulante Langzeitrehabilitation nach Myocardinfarkt. Deutsche Med Wochenschr 101:674

Mulcahy R (1982) Do different kinds of social and cultural settings require different kinds of rehabilitation programs? In: Mathes P, Halhuber M (eds) Controversies in cardiac rehabilitation. Springer, Berlin Heidelberg New York, p 140

Oberwittler W, Schulte H (1975) Untersuchungen über die Spätletalität nach Myocardinfarkt. Med Welt 28:2018

Stocksmeier U, Stabl M, Natus W (1980) unpublished
Wenger NK, Hellerstein HK (1978) Rehabilitation of the coronary patient. John Wiley and
    Sons, New York Chichester Brisbane Toronto

Do Different Kinds of Social and Cultural Settings Require Different Kinds of Rehabilitation Programme?

R. Mulcahy

The frequency of coronary heart disease in Western communities, particularly amongst men during the active stages of life, makes it mandatory to have effective and feasible rehabilitation facilities available to all. These facilities should be provided irrespective of all social circumstances and of the material and professional resources available. In only exeptional circumstances are specialised rehabilitation facilities available and then mainly because of the interest and involvement of individual physicians and institutions, and the availablity of exceptional financial resources.

At. St. Vincent's Hospital, Dublin, we have adopted a cardiac rehabilitation programme which has consistently enabled us over a period of 15 years to return 90% of survivors of myocardial infarction under 60 years to work. Nearly all our patients return to full-time normal employment and job changes are seldom prescribed.

Our approach to rehabilitation can be described as an informal and modest one, and is based on the limited personnel normally available in a large district teaching hospital. It is therefore designed to function in a situation where there are limited financial and material resources. The rehabilitation programme is organized and supervised by a small team made up of two cardiologists, a social worker, a physiotherapist, a psychologist, a dietitian and the nurses in the coronary care unit and in the rehabilitation clinic. With the exception of the social worker, all members of the team devote only part of their time to rehabilitation work.

The design of the programme has not changed substantially over the past 10 years although the work has been facilitated by a grant from the European Social Fund since 1978. The purpose of the grant is to enable us to communicate our techniques of rehabilitation to outside practitioners and hospitals in an endeavour to provide optimum rehabilitation for heart cases in our country.

Our rehabilitation policy is based on the following principles:

1. Early ambulation after admission to the coronary care unit, early discharge from hospital and early return to work.

   All patients in the coronary care unit, except those with obvious severe complications, are encouraged to get out of bed and to start graduated walking exercise within 24 h of the cessation of pain. The average stay in hospital for our patients is 9 days with the uncomplicated good risk cases being discharged in 6—7 days.

2. Risk factor intervention. Patients are encouraged to change their lifestyle and to cooperate fully in avoiding major coronary risk factors. Risk factor intervention is carried out through detailed interviews with the patient and by providing special booklets in an effort to explain the importance of cooperation in this area.

3. Individualised home exercise programme. Patients are advised to start a walking programme as soon as they return home. They are encouraged to walk up to 3 miles (5 km) daily by the time of the first return visit to the rehabilitation clinic 3 weeks after discharge. The patient's preferences, inclinations and opportunities are of course considered in prescribing an exercise programme. All forms of exercise which are not competitive

or excessively vigorous are encouraged and ideally we encourage patients to walk about three miles every day.

4. Conservative approach to medication and coronary artery by-pass surgery. Routine use of beta-blockers, anticoagulants, calcium antagonists and longterm nitrates is discouraged and coronary artery by-pass surgery is prescribed only in patients who suffer from disabling angina or who manifest other clinical and investigational evidence of advanced chronic obstructive disease of the coronary arteries. In fact, disabling angina is relatively rare amongst our patients if they follow risk factor advice and exercise programmes as indicated.

5. Regular visits to rehabilitation clinic. Patients are encouraged to visit the clinic 3 weeks, 3 months and a further 6 months after the coronary event. They are subsequently encouraged to visit the clinic every 6 months or 1 year depending on their need for advice and encouragement.

6. No group or institutional training is prescribed.

7. Stress test, coronary arteriography and other complex investigations are employed selectively and only according to well-defined limited criteria.

8. All major investigations or major therapeutic interventions are avoided if at all possible during the convalescent stage. Such interventions are performed when necessary early after discharge or after the patient has returned to work. The full psychological, physical and social rehabilitation of patients can be considerably delayed by interventions which may be dragged out during a prolonged convalescent phase.

Results

The results of our rehabilitation programme were first presented at the International Society of Cardiology Meeting in London in 1970 [1]. A second communication was made at the meeting on psychological factors in the rehabilitation of coronary patients in Höhenried in 1974 [2]. Our programme is principally aimed at returning patients to a normal life and to normal work. Our success in returning patients to work has not changed materially over the last 15 years.

The present report deals with 197 successive patients under 60 years who were admitted to the coronary care unit between 1st February 1978 and 31st January 1980. These patients have been followed for at least 1 year. Follow-up information is inadequate in three, leaving 194 subjects for analysis: 163 male and 31 female. All had been admitted to hospital with fresh unstable angina or myocardial infarction. Seventy-five per cent had returned to work within 3 months of the onset of their illness and this figure had increased to 92% at last follow-up. This figure includes three subjects who were working part-time. All the women had returned to work by the end of the period of observation and 90% of the men had returned to work.

Fourteen patients were unemployed at entry. Twelve of these eventually returned to work. We attributed this unexpectedly good result to the enthusiasm and perseverance of our social worker and of other members of the team, and to our close and active relationship with employers, and with retraining and reemployment agencies.

Analysis of the early return to work data confirm that there were four determinants of delayed return to work. They included:

1. Unemployment before the initial attack
2. A severe initial attack with left ventricular failure or other serious complication
3. Angina of effort at follow up
4. Poor motivation as assessed by psychological testing.

However, Table 1 confirms that these four determinants of delayed return to work no longer operated at the end of the period of observation. By then there was no statistical difference in the return to work status of the patients, irrespective of unemployment before the illness, the severity of the initial attack, the presence of post-infarction angina or bad motivation as measured by psychological testing. It appears therefore that a prolonged personalised and multidisciplinary rehabilitation approach to patients will succeed, even with subjects endowed with unfavourable rehabilitation attributes.

Table 2 confirms the influence of the method of rehabilitation on a number of factors closely involved with the rehabilitation process.

It can be seen that informal individualised rehabilitation at home is particularly appropriate in relation to cost, applicability, longterm acceptability and flexibility. Applicability refers to its suitability for most hospital and communities where there are limited resources as regards money and personnel avaiable. Apart from these advantages we have no reason to believe that home exercise programmes are associated with increased risk of serious arrhythmias or fresh infarction.

Conclusion

An informal approach to the rehabilitation of coronary patients has been succesful over a 15-year period in circumstances of limited financial and material resources. The success of this programme can be attributed to the following factors:

1. The involvement of a small dedicated team made up of personnel attached to the normal cardiac service of the hospital
2. The continued involvement of the cardiologist who attends the patients during their initial illness in the coronary care unit
3. The provision of a follow-up clinic where patients are seen regularly and where they are encouraged to attend at least once a year after their full rehabilitation

Table 1. Determinants of return to work

	No.	RTW[a]	%
1. Employed at entry	180	167	92.8
Unemployed	14	12	85.7
2. Uncomplicated attack	122	115	94.3
Complicated attack	72	64	88.9
3. No angina at follow-up	104	96	92.3
Angina at follow-up	90	83	92.3
4. Good motivation[b]	154	142	92.2
Bad motivation	27	25	92.6

[a] RTW, Return to work
[b] Psychological assessment inadequate in 13 subjects

Table 2. Factors to consider when assessing rehabilitation and physical training programmes

Factors		Home	Out-patient	In-patient
Efficacy	Fitness	+	++	++
	Involvement	++	++	++
Safety		+	++	++
Expense		+	++	+++
Applicability		+++	+	+
Longterm acceptability		+++	+	−
Flexibility		+++	++	++
Adverse effects on rehabilitation		−	+	+

4. Emphasis on risk factor intervention and on an adequate exercise and a physical fitness programme
5. Good communication between the rehabilitation team and relatives, employers, and employment and retraining agencies

References

1 Mulcahy R, Hickey N (1970) The rehabilitation of patients with coronary heart disease. Scand J Rehab Med 2/3:108
2 Mulcahy R (1977) The rehabilitation of patients with coronary heart disease: A clinician's view. In: Stocksmeier U (ed) Psychological approach to the rehabilitation of coronary patients. Springer, Berlin Heidelberg New York

Stress Testing

B. Carù

Effort Angina

In case of effort angina a test will be effective if it is able to increase myocardial oxygen consumption to prove an inadequate increase in myocardial blood flow.

In our experience dynamic exercise is the most reliable test for effort angina [1]. Its sensitivity is directly proportional to the degree of coronary involvement. Our experience is shown in more detail in Table 1.

With a careful statistical quantitative analysis made in our department on 480 patients who underwent coronary angiography [2], the quantitative response of the exercise test in terms of ST down-sloping, type of down-sloping, duration of ST down-sloping and occurence of angina was dependent on the degree of coronary artery involvement, as shown in Table 1.

In effort angina our experience was completely unsatisfactory with atrial pacing [3]. This type of stress test, in our hands, showed a sensitivity of 55%. Equally unsatisfactory, in our experience, is the isometric exercise test in patients with effort angina [4]. We found a low sensitivity when we subjected patients with pure effort angina to the cold pressor test (CPT) [5].

Data from Lassvik and Areskog [6] show that exposure to cold causes a rapid physiological response in man. The main effect is cutaneous vasoconstriction, with an increase in the peripheral resistance and the systemic blood pressure. With shivering, and with intense acute cooling, an increase in the cardiac output is induced. Coronary resistance may increase in patients with ischemic heart disease. During exercise the hemodynamic changes induced by cooling may be counterbalanced by muscular vasodilatation.

Table 1. Sensitivity of dynamic exercise electrocardiography in detecting coronary artery disease

1 V	59%	2 V	81%	3 V	94%
RC	42	RC + Cx	78		
Cx	51	Cx + LAD prox	88		
LAD prox	88	RC + LAD prox	89		
LAD dist	60				

Angina at Rest

In angina at rest, the mechanism does not involve an increase in myocardial oxygen consumption. From a theoretical point of view the stress tests which increase that parameter should not be effective in the diagnostic prodecure of this disease. In connection with angina at rest it was clearly proven that the occurrence of coronary spasm is the determinant factor of the anginal attack .

In fact in our experience the dynamic exercise in patients with angina et rest showed a poor effectiveness [8]. Recent data maintain a higher sensitivity of the dynamic test if it is performed early in the morning, and this is probably due to a different response of the autonomic nervous system [9].

Atrial pacing, both in angina at rest and in effort angina, is a test of poor effectiveness in provoking symptoms useful for diagnostic purposes. The isometric stress test, as is well known, causes a considerable increase of blood pressure and a lower increase of heart rate; it was not satisfactory in our hands if applied to patients with angina at rest [10].

Among the tests that could provoke spasm, the CPT is really effective. Raizner and co-workers showed by means of quantitative coronary angiography that the luminal diameter of normal coronary segments significantly decreases in response to cold pressor stimulation [11]. Patients who are prone to coronary spasm may represent one extreme of a spectrum of reactivity to a coronary vasoconstrictive stimulus.

The CPT can provoke focal coronary artery spasm in certain patients and may be a useful nonpharmocologic provocative test to aid in the diagnosis of this phenomenon. Hemodynamic measurements showed a significant increase of aortic systolic pressure, while heart rate did not change significantly. An easily performed and safe provocative test that does not require the administration of pharmacologic agents whould be of value in attempting to provoke coronary artery spasm, particularly in patients with coronary artery disease. The CPT is relatively simple to perform, and the response to cold occurs rapidly and is readily reversed by discontinuing the cold stimulus and administration of nitroglycerin.

Cold pressor stimulation induces reflex vasoconstriction of multiple vascular beds with a consequent increase in peripheral vascular resistance and systemic arterial blood pressure. The CPT provokes generalized coronary vasoconstriction in most patients and can provoke focal spasm of the coronary vasculature in some. Focal spasm often occurs primarily in the vicinity of atheromatous disease. Thus, a negative CPT does not exlude the diagnosis of spontaneous angina.

The observations of Lassvik and Areskog [6] previously mentioned show that exposure to a cold environment or cold air inhalation, probably by similar mechanisms as in the CPT, is an affective provocative factor in patients with angina at rest. It is unquestionable that the ergonovine test is particularly effective as a provocative test for coronary artery spasm [12].

In Table 2 our own experience is summarized and data from the literature on the effectiveness of different stress tests in different forms of angina are given.

Table 2. Usefullness of different stress tests in the various forms of angina

	Dynamic exercise	Atrial pacing	Isometric exercise	CPT	Cold	Ergonov.
Effort angina	+++	–	–	–	+ –	+ –
Angina at rest	+ –	–	+ –	++	++	+++
Effort and rest A	++	–	+ –	++	++	++

References

1   De Vita C, Ciliberto GR, Gibelli G, Caru B (1977) Contributo della prova alla diagnostica dell'angina da sforzo stabile tipica. G Ital Cardiol 7:1047
2   Caru B, Pirelli S, Candotti C, Catafi G, Manzini A (1979) Interpretazione quantitativa delle prove da sforzo. In: Pozzi L (ed) Aggiornamenti in cardiologia. Roma
3   De Ponti C, Gibelli G, Caru B, Rovelli F (1976) L'atrial pacing nella diagnosi di insufficienza coronarica. Atti VII Congresso Nazionale ANMCO, Firenze, 1976
4   Caru B, de Ponti C (1979) Isometric stress test in coronary patients. In: Rossi P (ed) Functional evaluation and rehabilitation on cardiac patients. Novara
5   Caru B, Pirelli S, Gasparini M, de Biase AM (to be published) Cold pressor test in effort and spontaneous angina
6   Lassvik C, Areskog NH (1979) Angina pectoris in cold environment – Reactions to exercise. Br Heart J 39:512
7   Maseri A (1979) Pathophysiology of coronary spasm. In: Kelly DT (ed) Variant angina – Diagnosis and treatment. Melbourne
8   Caru B, Knippel M, de Ponti C (1976) La prova da sforzo nell'angina spontanea. In: Pozzi L (ed) Attulita in cardiologia. Roma
9   Hirofumi Y, Shingo O, Akinori T, Massao N, Kamihisa M, Satoru T: Circadian variation of exercise capacity in patients with Prinzmetal's Variant angina: role of exercise induced coronary arterial spasm
10 Caru B, Figini A, Bechi G (1976) Valutazione comparativa dello sforzo isometrico e del lavoro dinamico nella diagnosi dell'insufficienza coronarica. G Ital Cardiol 6:208
11 Raizner AE, Chahine RA, Ishimori T, Verani MS, Zacca N, Jamal N, Miller RA, Luchi RJ (1980) Provocation of coronary artery spasm by the cold pressor test. Hemodynamic, arteriographic, and quantitative angiographic observations. Circulation 62:925
12 Bernstein L (1979) Diagnostic use of ergonovine. In: Kelly DT (ed) Variant angina – Diagnosis and treatment. Melbourne
13 Guazzi M, Polese A, Fiorentini C, Magrini F, Olivari MT, Bartorelli C (1975) Left and right heart haemodynamics during spontaneous angina pectoris. Br Heart J 37:401
14 Angus J (1979) Alpha receptors in the coronary circulation. In: Kelly DT (ed) Variant angina – Diagnosis and treatment. Melbourne
15 Saxon White (1979) The neurogenic control of the circulation. In: Kelly DT (ed) Variant angina – Diagnosis and treatment. Melbourne
16 Bassan MM, Markus HS, Ganz W (1980) The effect of mild-to-moderate mental stress on coronary hemodynamics in patients with coronary artery disease. Circulation 62:933

Contribution of Nuclear Cardiology to the Diagnosis of the Various Stages of Coronary Artery Disease*

W.E. Adam, F. Bitter, and M. Stauch

Introduction

Nuclear cardiology claims to be able to contribute information on various aspects of myocardial diseases. The complete description of the myocardial state includes the perfusion, metabolism, and function of the myocardium. The immediate cause of myocardial disease is insufficient oxygen delivery, whereaus substrate delivery is not that important. The sensitivity of the system to very small perfusion defects results from the high extraction rate of oxygen, which in the myocardium reaches 75%; in normal muscle the extraction rate is only 25%. This is a critical point, because oxygen delivery cannot be effectively improved by an increase in extraction rate. Improvement is possible only by increasing the myocardial blood flow. Thus far, perfusion imaging is of paramount importance for detection of oxygen deficiency in the myocardium. Subsequent metabolic disorders, e.g., anaerobic glycolysis, call for their respective metabolic radionuclide indicators [1]. Finally, the metabolic failure results in functional abnormalities of the myocardium, which implies motion abnormalities (hypokinesis, dyskinesis), which can be visualized by radionuclide ventriculography.

In summary, nuclear cardiology means imaging of myocardial perfusion (perfusion scintigraphy), visualization of myocardial metabolism (metabolism scintigraphy), and detection of regional wall motion abnormalities (RWMA) by radionuclide ventriculography (wall motion scans, parametric scans). However, it should be made clear that these procedures include quantitative data, e.g., volumes of the heart chambers and their time derivatives.

Imaging Procedures of Nuclear Cardiology

Imaging of myocardial perfusion yields information concerning substrate and oxygen delivery, whereas scintigraphy of metabolism means visualization of enegery storage and liberation (turnover). Finally, myocardial motion reflects energy utilization. This explains the high degree of interrelationship existing between the results of these three procedures.

Imaging of Myocardial Perfusion

The clinically most used indicator is thallium 201. Though metabolic factors also play a role in the distribution of the radionuclide, the predominant factor is indeed the perfusion. A linear relationship between the distribution of thallium 201 and blood flow in ischemic and nonischemic myocardium could be proven during rest conditions [2, 3] and during exercise [4]. Thallium 201 bears some resemblance to potassium. The uptake of both substances

---

* Dedicated to Prof. Dr. med. and Dr. rer. nat. E.H. Graul on his 60th birthday

into the cell is similar, due to their comparable ionic radius, which is an important determinant for the passive penetration of the cell membrane. Concentration in the viable myocardium depends on the blood level of thallium and on the concentration gradient which the viable cells can maintain. Since delivery to ischemic myocardium is limited, this tissue will require a longer time to reach the peak level than the nonischemic myocardium (redistribution effect). Nonviable myocardium in contrast will not accumulate thallium. So far, perfusion imaging is a valuable clinical tool in detecting coronary artery disease (CAD) and distinguishing between nonischemic, ischemic but viable, and infarcted myocardium [5].

Imaging of Myocardial Metabolism

Myocardial metabolism can be visualized by labeled physiologic substrates, which trace the metabolic pathways. Fluorine-18 2-deoxyglucose has been used as analog for glucose whereas long chain fatty acids labeled with iodine-123 have been applied for visualizing the fat metabolism. However, these procedures up to now have not gained broad clinical application.

Imaging of Myocardial Function (Motion)

Equilibrium (gated) radionuclide ventriculography is an analog to levocardiography, resulting in displaying the moving heart in cine mode [6]. Complete analysis of the data [7] results in a set of "parametric scans" for each patient, allowing a detailed analysis of regional wall motion abnormalities (Fig. 1).
Whereas tracing of myocardial metabolism up to now has not had significant impact on the clinical decision process, perfusion scintigraphy and radionuclide ventriculography have come to play an important role in the diagnostic process of CAD.

Definition of Stages of Coronary Artery Disease

Resting coronary flow and regional distribution are not affected by narrowing of up to 85% of arterial diameter and therefore provide little insight into the effects of stenoses on coronary hemodynamics. However, maximal coronary flow and coronary flow reserve are markedly reduced by constrictions that do not affect resting flow. Coronary flow reserve begins to decrease with stenosis of 30%–45% of arterial diameter [8]. Proudfit [9] assumed that 50% diameter stenosis in a coronary artery represents significant CAD. This was based on data from patients with angina and a positive ECG stress test. Taking into account these experimental and clinical data it seems appropriate to adapt the 50% limit as borderline between subcritical and significant coronary artery disease. Those patients with a 50% or greater reduction in luminal diameter in two or more coronary angiographic projections of one or more coronary arteries are considered to have significant coronary artery disease.
We are aware of the limitations of this definition, because it does not take into account site and length of the stenoses. A "coronary core" would better correspond to the real coronary state. However, for clinical purposes and listings of the literature, this seems roughly appropriate. "Subcritical stenoses" subsequently are defined by 25%–49% reduction in luminal diameter in two or more coronary angiographic projections of one or more coronary arteries.

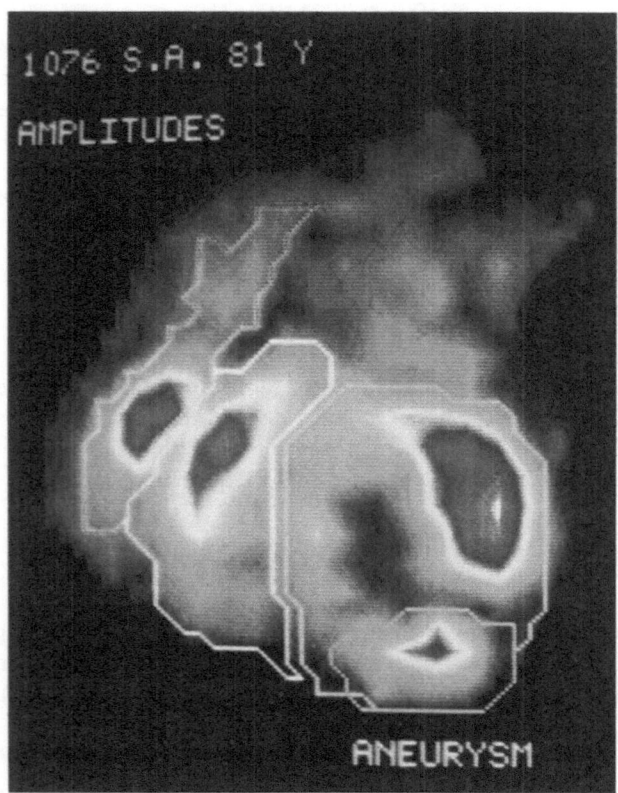

Fig. 1. Complete analysis of radionuclide ventriculography yields a set of "parametric scans," describing exactly regional wall motion abnormalities. The *"amplitude scan"* shows normokinectic (*red*) and hypokinetic (*blue-green*) regions. A large hypokinetic area extends from the base to the LV apex

"No coronary stenoses" includes subjects with reduction of the diameter less than 25%. The group "significant stenoses" comprises stable angina and unstable angina. The subsequent sections deal with contributions of myocardial perfusion scintigraphy and myocardial motion scintigraphy (radionuclide ventriculography) to the diagnosis of CAD, ranging from stage I to IV:

Stage I: Subcritical stenosis
Stage II: Significant stenosis
Stage III: Myocardial infarction
Stage IV: Postinfarction state

Contribution of Nuclear Cardiology to the Diagnosis of Subcritical Stenoses

Pohost et al. [5] found that 12 of 18 patients with subcritical CAD (20%–49% narrowing) had one or more defects on their initial postexercise thallium imaging study. Only one of

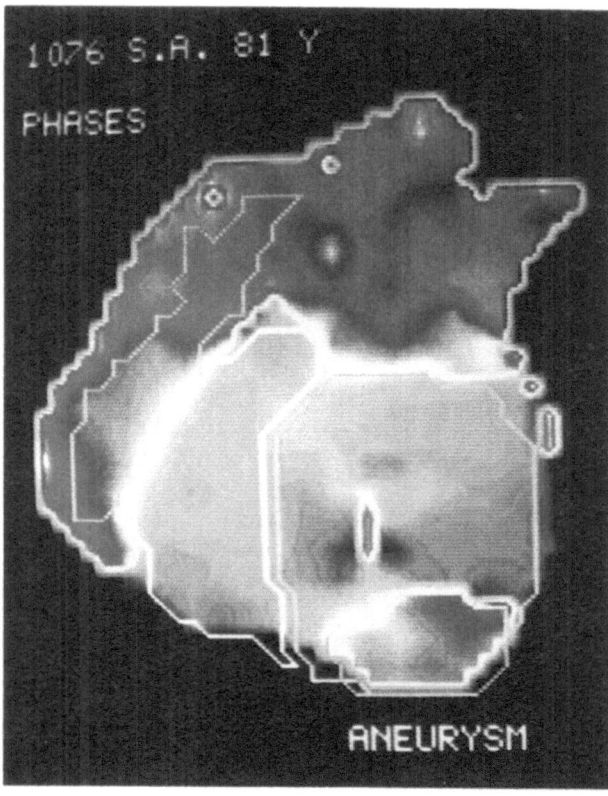

Fig. 2. The "phase scan" additionally detects a dyskinetic (*red*) region in the LV apex. *Diagnosis:* Hypokinesis of the anterior LV wall and apical aneurysm

the patients had typical angina. These findings illuminate the special value of the perfusion scans: While angina pectoris and ECG changes are associated with functional ischemia, the thallium 201 study depends only upon the presence of inhomogenous flow and not on the presence of functional ischemia. However, a real estimate of the predictive value in diagnosing subcritical stenoses up to now is not possible.

Contribution of Nuclear Cardiology to the Diagnosis of Significant Stenoses

The thallium exercise test (TET) in patients with significant stenoses is now accepted as being more reliable than the exercise ECG (EECG). The sensitivity in various independent groups ranges between 75% and 99% (as compared with EECG 61%–79%) and the specificity between 69% and 90% (EECG 69% and 82%) (Table 1). The superiority of the TET becomes especially clear in single vessel disease (SVD): The sensitivity was 73% versus 43% (EECG). Stenosed coronary arteries with angiographically proven collaterals yielded TET defects in only 65 of 92 patients [13]. Of paramount interest is the "redistribution effect," which permits the differentiation of ischemic but viable myocardium from infarcted myo-

Table 1. Thallium-201 exercise tests: Significant coronary stenoses

	N	201 TL Sensit. %	Specific. %	ECG Sensit. %	Specific. %
1980 Pohost et al. [5] (Multiple Centers, USA)	1077	82	90	61	82
1980 Simoons and Hugenholtz [10]	118	75	86	59	76
1980 Sauer and Sebening [11]	120	91	94		
1980 Lösse and Loogen [12]	169	99	69	79	69
1981 Hör and Kanemoto [13] (Multiple Centers)	3092	83	90		

cardium. Activity in the normal myocardium reaches a peak within 10–20 min after injection and then leaves myocardium at a rate parallel to the blood. Accumulation in the ischemic region is very slow, but 2 h later has reached the level of the normal myocardium. In contrast, infarcted areas do not show a filling up of the defect. Variant or Prinzmetal's angina (coronary artery spasm with transmural ischemia) shows characteristic behavior: During the occlusion phase, thallium 201 kinetics in the ischemic zone resembles that of infarcted myocardium. After reflow, blood flow to previously ischemic myocardium becomes transiently hyperemic. Although blood flow is increased, the thallium 201 level in the blood is low. Accordingly, there is slow accumulation in the previously ischemic myocardium until it achieves a level equivalent to that in the nonischemic myocardium. Although late imaging may demonstrate total disappearance of defects (complete redistribution) after 2 h, sometimes the delay of redistribution may last up to 6 h. Perfusion defects have an immediate impact on ventricular function. Borer et al. [14] have shown a decrease of left ventricular ejection fraction (EF) and motion abnormality in the ischemic zone, whereas in normals EF increased. By this means differentiation of a normal and a CAD group with sensitivity and specificity of more than 90% was possible (Table 2).

These fascinating results could not be attained by other groups. Caldwell et al. [15] published results with a comparable sensitivity of 93%, but lower specificity of only 55%. Our own results revealed optimal sensitivity (100%) with poor specificity (54%), when "normal behavior" was defined as "increase of EF of more than 3%." In contrast, when "normal" was defined as "EF unchanged or increasing," specificity was increased to 85%, combined with a still good sensitivity of 84%. These results are comparable to those attained by TET. However, at the present state high sensitivity and lower specificity should be taken into account for radionuclide ventriculography with respect to detection of CAD. This gives high yield in detecting CAD in a population with high prevalence of this disease.

Best results of the RNV exercise test (RNVET) were obtained by regional wall motion analysis. The publication of Bodenheimer et al. [16] deserves special interest; they point out that qualitative evaluation of regional wall motion failed in detecting smaller abnormalities which could be revealed by the parametric scan procedure. The author applied the parameter "regional EF." This corresponds to our own experiences with presentation of "amplitude" and "phase" scintigraphy after Fourier analysis, though statistical proof is not

Table 2. Radionuclide ventriculography exercise tests: Signficant stenosis

	Sensitivity %	Specificity %	
Borer et al. [14]	94	91	Global EF
Bodenheimer et al. [16]	91	87	Reg. wall mot. (Ref) handgrip
Caldwell et al. [15]	93	55	Gobal EF
Nolan and Lindsay [17]	89	88	Reg. wall mot.
Sauer and Sebening [11]	83	100	Reg. wall mot.

available up to now. It is particularly interesting that the combination of "amplitude" and "phase" scans makes possible the delineation of the infarcted zone within the incoordinated contracting heart, e.g., in a case of left or right bundular branch block.

Contributions of Nuclear Cardiology to the Diagnosis of Myocardial Infarction

Though most acute myocardial infarctions offer no diagnostic problems in the coronary care unit, still a substantial group of patients remains with a questionable history and a non-diagnostic ECG. In these cases perfusion scintigraphy offers a highly valuable diagnostic tool. Wackers [18] could demonstrate that in the period within 6 h after onset all infarctions could be detected, irrespective of location, size, and whether transmural or nontransmural. The sensitivity decreased to 78% (transmural) and 52% (nontransmural) after 24 h. It should be mentioned that after this interval, positive infarction imaging with 99m technetium phosphate complexes can complement nuclear cardiology advantageously, but further discussion of that technique falls outside the scope of this paper.

The sensitivity of thallium-201 to detect acute myocardial infarctions was determined by Wackers in 200 consecutive patients with proven myocardial infarction. Overall, positive scans were obtained in 82%. Assessment of the infarction size was based on the SGOT level in the serum. Large infarctions were characterized by a level more than 3.5 times the upper limit of normal, and small infarctions by a level below 3.5 times the upper limit of normal. Large infarctions showed positive scans in 94% and small ones in only 57%. Nontransmural infarctions revealed a lower sensitivity of 63%, as compared with the 88% positive scans in transmural infarctions. It becomes evident that the fast decrease of sensitivity after 24 h limits the value of thallium-201 in detection and assessment of older myocardial infarctions. In our opinion, starting with the stage of infarction, RNV should become the prevalent diagnostic procedure for the following reasons:

1. Sensitivity of RNV is comparable in the first few hours after infarction and seems to become superior after 24 h: 89 consecutive patients admitted to our ward with suspected acute or older infarction were diagnosed by RNV. The correct diagnosis remained unknown to the nuclear physician. 77 patients revealed wall motion abnormalities. All of them finally were diagnosed as having infarction. This corresponds to a sensitivity for detection of myocardial infarction of 93%, whereas in all subjects without wall motion abnormalities further observation could rule out myocardial infarction (Table 3).

2. RNV allows assessment of myocardial function in terms of global LV parameters (e.g., LVEF, EDV) and of parametric scans with analysis of regional wall motion. Assessment

Table 3. Own results of RNV in 89 consecutive patients with suspected infarction

	Motion abnormality	No motion abnormality
Infarction clinically proven	77 (93%)	6
Infarction not clinically proven	0	6 (100%)

6 false negative
No false positive results

of resting myocardial function and follow-up of myocardial function are now of prior interest for the prognosis of the individual patient.

Contributions of Nuclear Cardiology in the Postinfarction Period

The ECG pattern of myocardial infarction is not helpful in predicting the prognosis of patients who have survived. Nontransmural infarctions may have a prognosis as poor as trans-

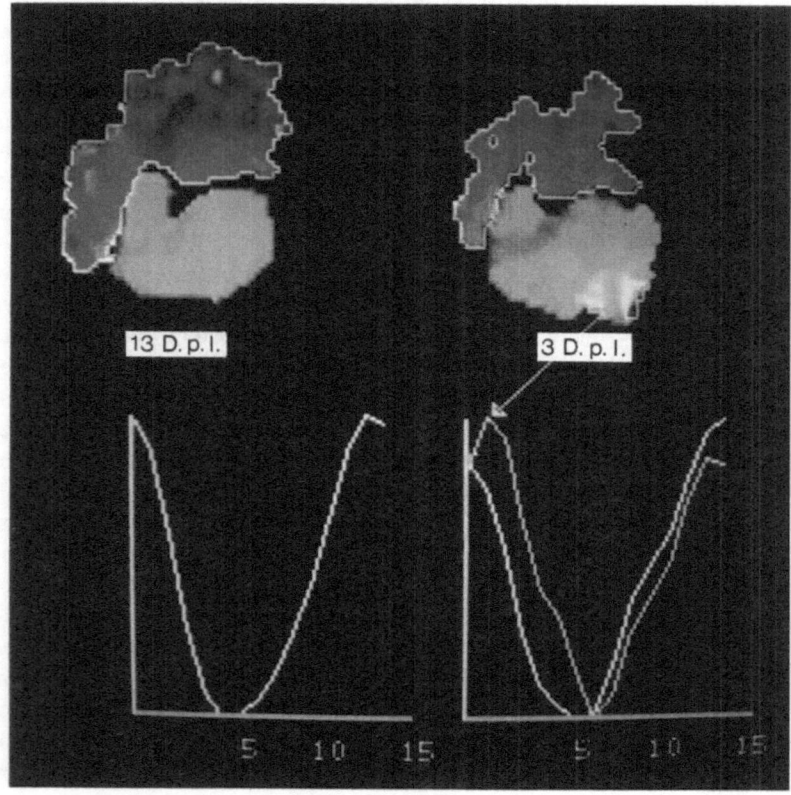

Fig. 3. Dyskinesis (*yellow*) of the latero-inferior LV wall 3 days after infarction. Complete normalization 10 days later

mural infarctions. Infarction may be a marker of CAD, but not necessarily an indicator of its severity. Taylor et al. [19] could demonstrate that low postinfarction EF was associated with a high risk of sudden cardiac death. Multivariate analysis of 30 clinical and laboratory variables identified previous myocardial infarction and an EF less than 40% as the best predictors of mortality. All patients who died were identified by these two variables. Once the information of these two variables had been considered, neither three vessel disease nor complicated late hospital phase ventricular arrhythmias provided any additional information about mortality. EF, which can easily be obtained by RNV, thus far plays an important role in the rehabilitation phase after infarction. But this should remind us that EF is only a by-product of the far more informative imaging of *regional* myocardial motion, which can be assessed in a quantitative manner, or in a semiquantitative way by parametric scanning. This yields the unique possiblity of follow-up studies of postinfarction RWMA in the individual patient. The divergent development of a dyskinesis in two patients after infarction is shown in Figs. 3 and 4. Three days after infarction, outward bulging of the anterolateral wall of the LV is evident. The time-activity (time-volume) curve of this region shows a delay of motion of 15% of the total heart cycle. Ten days later complete normalization of the myocardial motion is evident with good prognosis. In contrast, the second patient (Fig. 4) reveals im-

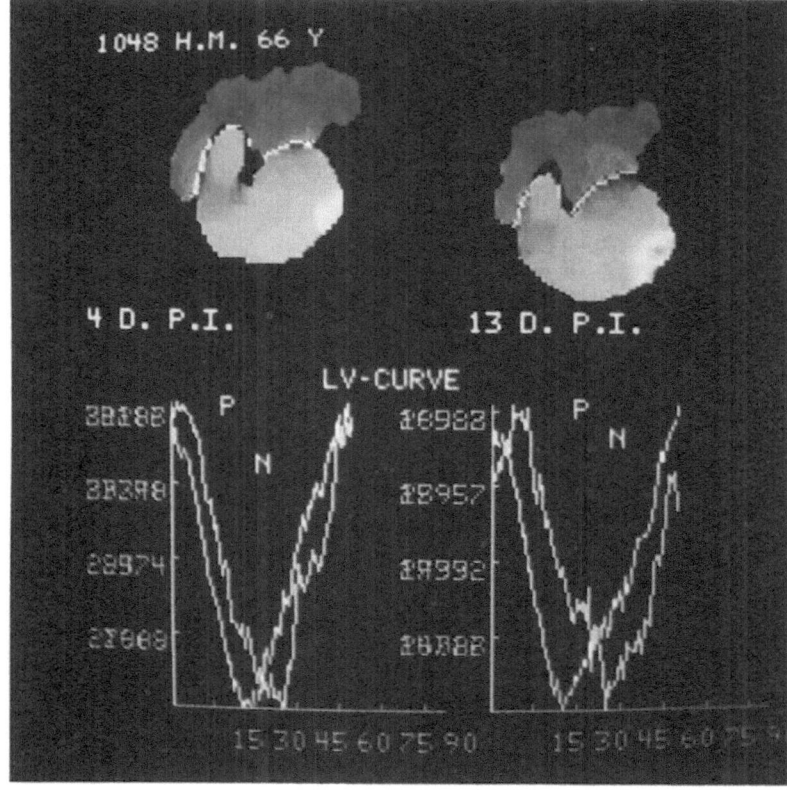

Fig. 4. Dyskinesis after 3 days, comparable to Fig. 3, but further impairment 10 days later. Imminent aneurysm possible. *N,* normal LV; *P,* dyskinetic region

pairment of the dyskinesis with increasing size of the abnormal region and further delay of the motion.

In conclusion, nuclear cardiology may contribute considerably to all stages of CAD. Whereas the stages of infarction and the postinfarction area are the domain of RNV, especially in the more sophisticated presentation of parametric scanning, thallium scans are preferably applied to the preinfarction stages of CAD.

References

1 Schelbert HE, Phelps ME (1980) Physiologic tomography: A new means for the non-invasive measurement of myocardial metabolism, blood flow and function. Eur J Nucl Med 5:209
2 Mueller TM, Markus ML et al (1976) Limitations of thallium 201 myocardial perfusion scintigrams. Circulation 54:640
3 Gerwitz H et al (1978) The affect of ischemia on thallium 201 clearance from the myocardium. Circulation 58:215
4 Nielsen AP et al (1980) Linear relationship between the distribution of thallium 201 and blood flow in ischemic and nonischemic myocardium during exercise. Circulation 61:797
5 Pohost GM et al (1980) Thallium redistribution: Mechanisms and clinical utility. Semin Nucl Med 10:70
6 Strauss HW et al (1971) A scintiphotographic method for measuring left ventricular ejection fraction in man without catherization. Am J Cardiol 28:575
7 Adam WE et al (1979) Equilibrium (gated) radionuclide ventriculography. Cardiovasc Radiol 2:161
8 Gould KL, Lipscomb K (1974) Effects of coronary stenoses on coronary flow reserve and resistance. Am J Cardiol 34:48
9 Proudfit WL, Shirey LK, Sones FM (1966) Selective cine coronary angiography: Correlation with clinical findings in 1000 patients. Circulation 33:901
10 Simons ML, Hugenholtz PG (1980) Value and limitations of exercise testing in coronary artery disease. Proceed. Int. Symposion Dubrovnik
11 Sauer E, Sebening H (1980) Myokard- und Ventrikelszintigraphie, Mannheim
12 Loogen F, Lösse B (1980) Comparative study between thallium scintigraphy and coronary angiography. Proceed. Int. Sympoion Dubrovnik
13 Hör G, Kanemoto N (to be published) 201 TI scintigraphy: Current status in coronary artery disease. Nucl Med
14 Borer JS et al (1977) Real time radionuclide cineangiography in the non ivasive evaluation of global and regional left ventricular function at rest and during exercise in patients with coronary artery disease. N Engl J med 296:839
15 Caldwell JH, Hamilton GW et al (1980) The detection of coronary artery disease with radionuclide techniques: A comparison of rest exercise thallium imaging and ejection fraction response. Circulation 61:610
16 Bodenheimer MM et al (1979) Comparison of wall motion and regional ejection fraction at rest and during isometric exercise. J Nucl Med 20:724
17 Nolan NG, Lindsay J (1980) The radionuclide cardiac ventriculogram. Eur J Nucl Med 407–410
18 Wackers FJ (1980) Myocardial imaging in the coronary care unit. The Hague Boston London
19 Taylor GJ et al (1980) Predictors of clinical course, coronary atomy and left ventricular function after recovery from acute myocardial infarction. Circulation 62:960

Echocardiography in Coronary Artery Disease

R.S. Meltzer, J. Roelandt, and P.G. Hugenholtz

Introduction

The complications of acute myocardial infarction where echocardiography can play an important role are listed in Table 1. Echocardiography is especially important in assessing anatomic complications such as aneurysms, thrombus, papillary muscle rupture, and ventricular septal defect. The technique is applicable at the bedside and this is important since there is reluctance to subject patients with acute infarction to catheterization. Some of the complications listed in Table 1 have surgical implications, and it is thus frequently useful to have a rapid and safe noninvasive method of confirming or making the diagnosis.

Acute Complications of Infarction

Both M-mode and two-dimensional echocardiography are sensitive methods of assessing left ventricular function [1–3]. Furthermore, two-dimensional echocardiography can assess local myocardial contractility and the state of the entire left ventricle in most patients [4–5]. Two-dimensional echocardiography has an advantage over M-mode echo in that it can assess apical and lateral wall motion of the left ventricle, while M-mode can examine the cardiac base alone. The pathology in coronary disease is often apical.

Pump Failure

Hypotension in the setting of acute infarction has multiple etiologies. If it is not caused by a dysrhythmia, it may be due to hypovolemia, tamponade, mechanical problems such

Table 1. Complications of myocardial infarction where echo may be useful

I. Acute
   1. Poor pump function
   2. Rupture ⟨ Free wall
                      Interventricular septum
   3. Mitral regurgitation ⟨ Papillary muscle dysfunction
                                Flail mitral leaflet
   4. Right ventricular infarction
II. Chronic
   1. Aneurysm ⟨ Subacute regional LV dilatation
                    True aneurysm
                    False or pseudo-aneurysm
   2. Left ventricular thrombi
   3. Pericardial effusion

as VSD or mitral regurgitation, or primary myocardial failure. These entities may be differentiated echocardiographically, and myocardial failure from regional aneurysmal dilatation may also be distinguished from more global dysfunction due to "ischemic cardiomyopathy." We have several times been called to the coronary care unit to evaluate a patient in cardiogenic shock who was thought to have primary myocardial dysfunction but echocardiographically had a normal-size left ventricle and hyperactive motion of at least a part of the left ventricle. These patients have either ventricular septal defects or mitral regurgitation, with soft or non-existent murmurs due to low output, frequently masked by the noise from the various apparatus of a modern coronary care unit – balloon pump, respirators, etc.

Patients with hypotension due to VSDs or mitral regurgitation from papillary muscle rupture always have hyperkinetic hearts. These are easy to differentiate from the grossly dilated hypocontractile heart of a patient with primary pump failure due to myocardial infarction. Cardiac tamponade is a rare complication of infarction, sometimes due to free wall rupture, rarely to catheter perforation, and occasionally related to the same disease process that caused the infarction – aortic root dissection, uremia, collagen-vascular diseases. In these cases pericardial effusion is present, though specific echocardiographic diagnosis of tamponade is diffficult and tamponade remains a clinical diagnosis [6–9].

Acute Mitral Regurgitation

Acute mitral regurgitation may complicate myocardial infarction via two different mechanisms with similar causes. That is, the papillary muscle may be dysfunctional, especially in inferior infarctions, and cause mitral regurgitation mainly late in systole due to its lack of contraction [10]. The same area may also rupture and cause flail mitral leaflet. The first condition may also progress the second. The echocardiographic hallmark of flail mitral leaflet is classically a systolic echo in the left atrium which disappears during diastole, and frequently a picture of accentuated holosystolic prolapse in the M-mode tracing at the mitral level. The diagnosis is by no means always so simple, however, and flail mitral leaflet can closely simulate a left atrial myxoma or mitral mass. Two-dimensional echocardiography can more reliably differentiate these conditions than can M-mode. This difference is usually apparent from the clinical setting, however. Papillary muscle dysfunction is recognized on M-mode echocardiography by a largely intact mitral apparatus. Recent abstracts have suggested that papillary muscle dysfunction can be recognized on two-dimensional echocardiography by abnormal mitral leaflet coaptation, but we have serious reservations about the reliability of this sign. Further confirmation will be required before papillary muscle dysfunction becomes an echocardiographic diagnosis.

Though two-dimensional echocardiography can frequently detect associated conditions in mitral regurgitation and thereby help elucidate its etiology and significance [11], we are currently witnessing early studies of another technique which promises th yield important and clinically useful information about mitral regurgitation in the future: pulsed Doppler echocardiography [12]. Doppler echocardiography can directly detect and perhaps eventually quantify the extent and severity of the mitral regurgitation [13, 14]. The problems with this approach are largely technical: it has been difficult to create a "duplex" instrument with coordinated and reliable two-dimensional images and an operator-directed volume sample for pulsed Doppler signals. Also, the physical limitations of the pulsed Doppler method are such that the higher velocity jets of either mitral or aortic regurgitation cannot be quantified in real time at the depths necessary in adult echocardiographic work. Parenthetically, this may not be the case in infants, where a shorter transducer-to-target distance allows more frequent sampling of the Doppler signal.

Laboratories testing new clinical Doppler equipment are currently trying to map the extent of mitral regurgitation in time and space within the left atrium — and even pulmonary veins.

Perhaps new developments such as color-coded Doppler echocardiography using digital multigate techniques [15, 16], or the application of fast Fourier transform chips to allow real-time Doppler signal quantification, will improve our ability to yield clinically useful information in mitral regurgitation in the future. As with many advances in echocardiography, by the way, the current industrial development of fast Fourier analysis represents a civilian application of technology developed for the military.

Ventricular Rupture

Left ventricular free wall rupture is usually immediately fatal, though several cases have been diagnosed ante mortem in Rotterdam using the commercially available MiniVisor (Organon Teknika) [17].

Ruptures of the interventricular septum are a complication of myocardial infarction that may be survived and are important to diagnose, since they lead to an abrupt worsening of hemodynamics. Classically this diagnosis is made due to the new presence of a holosystolic murmur, frequently heard better at the sternal border than axilla, and significant increases in oxygen saturation from the right atrium to pulmonary artery. Echocardiography can frequently visualize VSDs as "dropout" of echoes in the interventricular septum, though this sign is unreliable due to its poor sensitivity and specificity. A much better echocardiographic sign of intracardiac shunting is the detection of contrast crossing the septal defect [18, 19]. Unlike ASDs, where the large majority of shunts can be detected by peripheral venous injections, VSDs are often not detected by right-to-left shunting after peripheral vein injections. This is one of the reasons why our group [20, 21] and others [22] are interested in the possibilities of transmission of echocardiographic contrast through the lungs. We are currently studying microbubble dynamics and their removal by the lungs [23, 24], with the goal of developing noninvasive and safe methods of transmission of ultrasonic contrast through the lungs. If this can be obtained, the echocardiographic diagnosis of VSDs using contrast echocardiography to image left-to-right shunts may be improved.

Right Ventricular Infarction

At present right ventricular infarction is usually diagnosed by hemodynamic or scintigraphic techniques. It can occasionally be suspected or diagnosed echocardiographically by finding a dilated hypocontractile right ventricle, sometimes associated with "paradoxical" interventricular septal motion in the absence of septal infarction. The right ventricle is best examined by two-dimensional echocardiography in the parasternal and apical four-chamber views.

Chronic Complications of Myocardial Infarction

Aneurysm

Though M-mode echocardiography can show local dyskinesis and suggest the presence of a left ventricular aneurysm [25—27], it was only with the advent of two-dimensional echocardiography that noninvasive evaluation of patients for the presence of left ventricular aneurysms became a reality [28].

Echocardiography shares with angiography and radionuclide scintigraphy the disadvantage that localized dyskinesis does not always imply that a surgeon will find a discrete aneurysm at operation. Echocardiography does have an advantage over the other two techniques, however, in that it can not only image endocardial wall motion but also assess local left ventricular wall thickening. A true aneurysm has a thin wall which does not thicken during systole and often actually thins. Using quantitative techniques such as that of Eaton et al. [29], it may even be possible to diagnose echocardiographically those patients at risk for aneurysm development due to semiacute infarct expansion.

Due to the noninvasive nature of this technique, all patients with persistent ST elevation on ECG after infarction or with other clinical signs of possible aneurysm (difficult to control failure of ventricular dysrhythmias, prolonged apical impulse on physical examination) should have two-dimensional echocardiographic evaluation for the possibility of a ventricular aneurysm.

Pseudoaneurysm

A pseudoaneurysm is a more dangerous complication of myocardial infarction than a true left ventricular aneurysm, because its natural history is rupture and death and its detection frequently should be followed by an operation. One of the first uses uf two-dimensional echocardiography reported from our institution was the detection of a left ventricular pseudoaneurysm in 1975 [30]. At that time two-dimensional echocardiographic equipment developed at the Thoraxcenter and available to us was considerably more primitive than the equipment now commercially available. The important signs by which a pseudoaneurysm can be recognized include a smaller orifice size compared to maximal aneurysm dimension, sometimes the imaging of a discontinuity in the myocardial echo, and the lack of a clear-cut myocardial echo surrounding the aneurysm. Like true aneurysms, pseudoaneurysms exhibit dyskinetic motion and frequently harbor mural thrombi [31].

Left Ventricular Thrombi

Left ventricular thrombi are a frequent complication of myocardial infarction coming to autopsy [32] and about half of the chronic left ventricular aneurysms operated on at Stanford contain mural thrombi. The large majority of these thrombi are silent — that is, they never cause a clinically apparent embolus. Thus the natural history of left ventricular thrombus, and even its prevalence, is unknown. An important reason for this was the lack of a noninvasive screening test to diagnose left ventricular thrombi. Until the recent past, the only test for left ventricular thrombi was cardiac catheterization with left ventricular angiography, and even this is not always reliable and may miss even giant left ventricular mural thrombi [33].

This situation has changed in the past few years due to the introduction of two-dimensional echocardiography and the realization that it is a good, though by no means perfect, diagnostic test for left ventricular thrombi [34—36]. Two-dimensional echocardiography has unique characteristics that enhance its ability to detect left ventricular thrombi compared to the other widely used cardiac imaging techniques: its tomographic form of image processing allows display of different soft tissue characteristics at all point in its output, whereas angiography and scintigraphy integrate all information throughout the body thickness in the formation of their images. However, both false positive and false negative two-dimensional echocardiograms for left ventricular thrombi have been reported, and the interpretation of some studies requires considerable experience.

Pericardial Effusion

Dressler's syndrome is usually though not always associated with a pericardial effusion echocardiographically. The size of these effusions is usually small, and they can be detected using standard M-mode echocardiographic techniques [37—38].

Future Prospects

There are many exciting prospects for future developments in cardiac ultrasound, and we would like to end by sharing some of these with you.

1. Tissue Characterization

   Several groups are working on quantitative analysis of both reflected and transmitted ultrasonic signals with respect to frequency and amplitude characteristics. The ultimate aim of this sort of work is to quantitate the frequently observed echocardiographic observation that an infarcted, thin and fibrotic septum is often echocardiographically more dense than normal myocardium, that the abnormal hypertrophied myocardial tissue in IHSS seems to have a different "texture" from normal myocardium, that ultrasonic characterization of various types of liver pathology can often be made on the basis of the pattern of echoes returning from the hepatic parenchyma by experienced radiologists, etc. There have been several national conferences on this topic in the U.S. and interested readers are referred to the specialized literature [39—41].

2. Videodensitometric Processing of Contrast Two-Dimensional Echocardiographic Data to Obtain Indicator-Dilution Type Curves

   This work was originally reported by DeMaria and Bommer in abstract form in 1978 [42] and the group from the Mayo Clinic reported on similar techniques for shunt quantification soon thereafter [43]. Briefly, if one either holds a photoelectric cell in front of the video screen or uses a more complicated hardware and software setup to quantify video density within a given operator-designated area on a previously recorded video tape of a contrast injection, curves can be obtained such as that in Fig. 1. Bommer reported that the 50% and 90% decay time of these curves was correlated to cardiac output. Our analysis suggests that these curves may have an initial "overload" phase where the video-density is maximal and further contrast microbubbles in the heart are not reflected in in-

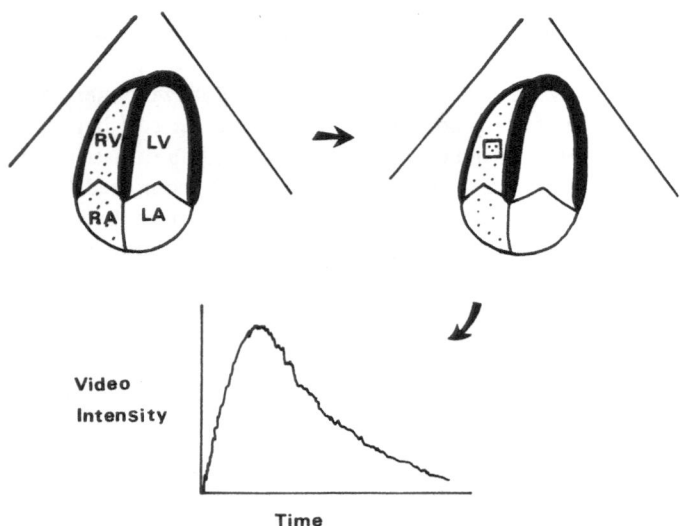

Fig. 1. Diagrammatic representation of method for obtaining videointensity versus time curves. *Upper left,* contrast appears in the right atrium (*RA*) and right ventricle (*RV*) during peripheral venous injection. *Upper right,* an area within the right ventricle is selected for analysis of video intensity within its boundaries. *Lower panel,* a curve (shown here as schematic representation) of videointensity versus time is thus obtained. *LV,* left ventricle, *LA,* left atrium

creased video-density. After this overload phase the decay is largely mono-exponential (unpublished data), as shown by a semilog plot of video-density versus time in Fig. 2. Indicator-dilution theory suggests that the decay phase of this curve may be used to quantify the relation between cardiac output and volume, or by using ECG gating may enable calculation of ejection fraction.

3. Presure Measurements Using Microbubble Resonant Frequencies

Since the resonant frequency of a microbubble of gas within the circulation is determined by its diameter (smaller bubbles have higher frequencies) and since the size of gas bubbles decreases with the ambient pressure in the fluid around them, the resonant frequency of microbubbles of contrast theoretically can be used to measure local pressure. Applying this theory has proven to be a very complex matter and has absorbed a good part of our energies over the past 2 1/2 years. Suffice it to say that this remains a theoretic possibility and only time will tell if pressures can practically be measured noninvasively with this method. The exciting point here is that perhaps in a time frame of about 5 years much of the information now available to the clinician only through Swan-Ganz pulmonary artery catherization (cardiac output, pulmonary pressures) may become available by a simple peripheral venous injection of microbubbles, with the help of a precordial echocardiographic instrument. Interested readers are referred to the annual reports of Rasor Associates, a small firm in Sunnyvale, California, which has developed this technology under contract from the National Heart, Lung, and Blood Institute [44].

4. Diagnosis of Proximal Coronary Narrowing

Here again is another exciting area of echocardiography where we are sure to see progress during the 1980s. The group from Indiana first reported imaging of a left main coronary

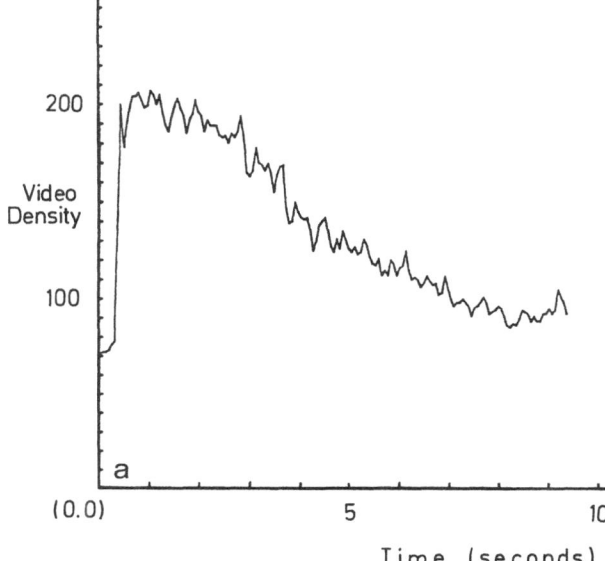

200

Video
Density

100

(0.0)   5   10

a

Time (seconds)

Fig. 2. a Actual videointensity curve obtained from computer analysis of the variation of videointensity within a surface area versus time. Videointensity units at the left are arbitrary

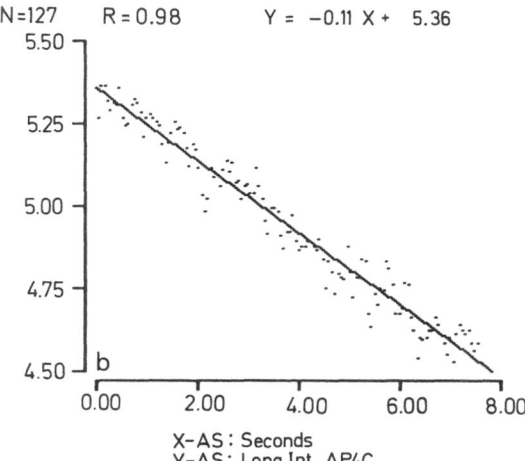

N=127   R=0.98   Y = −0.11 X + 5.36
5.50

5.25

5.00

4.75

4.50   b
0.00   2.00   4.00   6.00   8.00

X-AS : Seconds
Y-AS : Long.Int. AP4C

Fig. 2. b Semilogarithmic plot of the decay portion of the curve shown above. Ordinate is log videointensity. The linear decay here implies a mono-exponential decay of videointensity, as would be predicted theoretically

artery in 1976 [45]. At present, the left main coronary artery takeoff from the aorta can be imaged in the majority of patients. There has been great interest in the several reports claiming that two-dimensional echocardiography can be used, either with or without complex image processing techniques, to diagnose left main coronary disease [46, 47]. Although we agree that we can image the takeoff of the left and right coronary arteries from the sinuses of Valsalva in the majority of patients, we in Rotterdam do not feel that with present two-dimensional echocardiographic equipment proximal coronary stenosis can be reliably diagnosed. Part of the reason for this is that both the theoretic resolution capabilities of these instruments (based on wavelengths of 0.5 mm or so), and the measured resolution capabilities using test objects in vivo suggest that the ability to resolve "50%" from "70%" stenoses should not be expected from these machines. However, several developments now being implemented in our own engineering Division of Experimental Echocardiography as well as multiple commercial firms suggest that image quality will continue to improve in the 1980s. Part of this is simply the further implementation of the electronics revolution which has recently brought us miniaturized chip circuitry and many other developments. Part is due to new-generation design of echocardiographic equipment, incorporating triangulating compound scanning concepts, computed tomographic ideas, and many other more arcane developments which all promise to continue the betterment of images and decrease the cost of producing two-dimensional equipment at the same time.

We expect that the ultimate ability of echocardiography to make reliable diagnostic statements about the proximal coronary circulation will not be only due to improvement in resolving power due to the factors just mentioned, but also due to pulsed Doppler echocardiography and perhaps the transpulmonary transmission of echocardiographic contrast injected peripherally [20–22].

Conclusion

Many of the important complications of myocardial infarction can be readily detected by echocardiography. Since echocardiographic equipment is rapidly improving, we feel that an echocardiographic capability will be more and more helpful in the future both in the coronary care unit and in the out-patient treatment of patients with coronary artery disease. Echocardiography has developed largely during the past 5 years from a diagnostic technique frequently said to have little application in coronary disease to one where important information is available both clinically and for cardiovascular research in ischemic heart disease. Some of the developments outlined in the latter part of this article suggest that it will have an even greater impact in the 1980s and 1990s.

Acknowledgement. This work was done during the tenure of a Clinician-Scientist Award to Dr. Meltzer from the American Heart Association.

References

1 Popp RL (1977) Echocardiographic evaluation of left ventricular function. New Engl J Med 296:856
2 Meltzer RS, Popp RL (to be published) Echocardiographic analysis of left ventricular function. Indian Heart J
3 Roelandt J (1977) Practical echocardiology. Forest Grove, Oregon: Research Studies Press, Chapter 8: Assessment of left ventricular function, pp 117–136
4 Kisslo JA, Robertson D, Gilbert BW, von Ramm O, Behar VS (1977) A comparison of real-time, two-dimensional echocardiography and cineangiography in detecting left ventricular asynergy. Circulation 55:134
5 Bansal RC, Tajik AJ, Seward JB, Offord KP (1980) Feasibility of detailed two-dimensional echocardiographic examination in adults: Prospective study of 200 patients. Mayo Clin Proc 55:291
6 Schiller NB, Botvinick EH (1977) Right ventricular compression as a sign of cardiac tamponade. Circulation 56:774

7 Settle HP, Adolph RJ, Fowler NO et al (1977) Echocardiographic study of cardiac tamponade. Circulation 56:951
8 Horowitz MS, Schultz CS, Stinson EB et al (1972) Sensitivity and specifity of echo-cardiographic diagnosis of pericardial effusion. Circulation 50:239
9 Hancock EW (1979) Management of pericardial disease. Mod Concepts Cardiovasc Dis 48:1
10 Roberts WC, Perloff JK (1972) Mitral valvular disease. Ann Intern Med 77:939
11 Mintz GS, Kotler MN, Segal BL, Parry WR (1979) Two-dimensional echocardiographic evaluation of patients with mitral insufficiency. Am J Cardiol 44:670
12 Baker DW (1977) The present role of doppler techniques in cardiac diagnosis. Prog Cardiovasc Dis 21:517
13 Kalmanson D, Veyrat C, Bouchareine F, de Groote A (1977) Non-invasive recording of mitral value flow velocity patterns using pulsed Doppler echocardiography. Br Heart J 39:517
14 Abbasi AS, Allen MW, de Cristofaro D, Ungar I (1980) Detection and estimation of the degree of mitral regurgitation by range-gated pulsed Doppler echocardiography. Circulation 61:143
15 Brandestini M, Howard A, Eyer M, Stevenson J, Weiler T (1979) Visualization of intra-cardiac defects by M/Q mode echo: Doppler ultrasound. Circulation (Suppl II) 59–60: II–13
16 Stevenson G, Brandestini M, Weiler T, Howard A, Eyer M (1979) Digital multigate Doppler with color echo and Doppler display – diagnosis of atrial and ventricular septal defects. Circulation (Suppl II) 59–60: II–205
17 Hagemeijer F, Verbaan CJ, Sonke PCG, de Rooij CH (1980) Echocardiography and rupture of the heart. Br Heart J 43:45
18 Meltzer RS, Schwartz J, French J, Popp RL (1979) Ventricular septal defect noted by two-dimensional echocardiography. Chest 76:455
19 Scanlan JG, Seward JB, Tajik AJ (1979) Visualization of ventricular septal rupture utilizing wide-angle two-dimensional echocardiography. Mayo Clinic Proc 54:381
20 Meltzer RS, Serruys PW, McGhie J, Verbaan N, Roelandt J (1980) Pulmonary wedge injections yielding left sided echocardiographic contrast. Br Heart J 44:390
21 Meltzer RS, Sartorius OEH, Lancee CT, Serruys PW, Verdouw PD, Essed C, Roelandt J (1981) Transmission of echocardiographic contrast through the lungs. Ultrasound Med Biol 7:377
22 Reale A, Pizzuto F, Gioffre PA, Nigri A, Romeo F, Martuscelli E, Mangieri E, Scibilia G (1980) Contrast echocardiography, transmission of echoes to the left heart across the pumonary vascular bed. Eur Heart J 1:101
23 Meltzer RS, Tickner EG, Sahines TP, Popp RL (1980) The source of ultrasonic contrast effects. J Clin Ultrasound 8:121
24 Meltzer RS, Tickner EG, Popp RL (1980) Why do the lungs clear ultrasonic contrast? Ultrasound Med Biol 6:261
25 Kraemer R, Kerber RE, Abboud FM (1973) Ventricular aneurysm: Use of echocardio-graphy. J Clin Ultrasound 1:60
26 Dillon J, Feigenbaum H, Weyman AE et al (1976) M-mode echocardiography in the evaluation of patients for aneurysmectomy. Circulation 53:657
27 Petersen JL, Johnston W, Hessel EA, Murray JA (1972) Echocardiographic recognition of left ventricular aneurysm. Am Heart J 83:24
28 Weyman AE, Peskoe SM, Williams ES et al (1976) Detection of left ventricular aneurysm by cross-sectional echocardiography. Circulation 54:936
29 Eaton LW, Weiss JL, Bulkey BH, Garrison JB, Weisfeldt ML (1979) Regional cardiac dilatation after acute myocardial infarction. Recognition by two-dimensional echo-cardiography. N Engl J Med 300:57
30 Roelandt J, van den Brand M, Vletter WB, Nauta J, Hugenholtz PG (1975) Echocardio-graphic diagnosis of pseudo-aneurysm of the left ventricle. Circulation 52:466
31 Catherwood E, Mintz GS, Kotler MN, Parry WR, Segal BL (1980) Two-dimensional echocardiographic recognition of left ventricular pseudo aneurysm. Circulation 62:294

32   Garvin CF (1941) Mural thrombi in the heart. Am Heart J 21:713
33   Van Meurs H, Meltzer RS, van den Brand M, Essed CE, Michels HR, Roelandt J (1981) Illustrative echocardiogram: Superiority of echocardiography over angiography in diagnosing a left ventricular thrombus. Chest 80:321
34   Demaria AN, Bommer W, Neumann A, Grehl T, Weinart L, Denardo S, Amsterdam E, Mason DT (1979) Left ventricular thrombi identified by cross-sectional echocardiography. Ann Intern Med 90:14
35   Ports TA, Cogan J, Schiller NB, Rappaport E (1978) Echocardiography of left ventricular masses. Circulation 58:528
36   Meltzer RS, Guthaner D, Rakowski H, Popp RL, Martin RP (1979) Diagnosis of left ventricular thrombi by two-dimensional echocardiography. Br Heart J 42:261
37   Teicholz LE (1978) Echocardiographic evaluation of pericardial diseases. Prog Cardiovasc Dis 21:133
38   Horowitz MS, Schultz CS, Stinson EB, Harrison DC, Popp RL (1974) Sensitivity and specificity of echocardiographic diagnosis of pericardial effusion. Circulation 50:239
39   Linzer M (1976) Ultrasonic tissue characterization I. US Government Printing Office, Washington DC (National Bureau of Standards, Special Publication, No 453)
40   Linzer M (1979) Ultrasonic tissue characterization II. US Government Printing Office Washington DC (National Bureau of Standards, Special Publication, No 525)
41   Gramiak R, Waag RC, Schenk EA, Lee PPK, Thompson K, MacIntosch P (1979) Ultrasonic imaging of experimental myocardial infarcts. In: Lancee CT (ed) Echocardiology. Martinus Nijhoff, The Hague, pp 99−106
42   Bommer W, Neef J, Neumann A et al (1978) Indicator-dilution curves obtained by photometric analysis of two-dimensional echo-contrast studies (abstract). Am J Cardiol 41:370
43   Hagler DJ, Tajik AJ, Seward JB, Mair DD, Ritter DG, Ritman EL (1978) Videodensitometric quantitation of left-to-right shunts with contrast sector echocardiography (abstract). Circulation (Suppl II) 58: II−70
44   Tickner EG (1978) Noninvasive assessment of pulmonary hypertension using the bubble ultrasonic ringing pressure (BURP) method. National Institute of Health, Betheda (Report No HR-62917-2A)
45   Weyman AE, Feigenbaum H, Dillon JC, Johnston KW, Eggleton RC (1976) Non-invasive visualization of the left main coronary artery by cross sectional echocardiography. Circulation 54:169
46   Chen CC, Morganroth J, Ogawa S, Mardelli TJ (1980) Detecting left main coronary artery disease by apical, cross-sectional echocardiography. Circulation 62:238
47   Chandrarathna PAN, Aronow WS (1980) Left main coronary arterial patency assessed with cross-sectional echocardiography. Am J Cardiol 46:91

Towards the Optimal Lead System and Optimal Criteria for Exercise Electrocardiography*

M.L. Simoons and P. Block

Summary

In order to define the optimal lead system for exercise electrocardiography, data are analyzed of the whole body-surface potential distribution at rest and during exercise in 25 normal subjects and in 25 patients with coronary artery disease. All patients had a normal electrocardiogram at rest.
Sensitivity of the standard chest leads was 60%; it improved to 84% with the body surface map while both methods had a 100% specificity. Based on these data, and reports from other centers, it is concluded that a single bipolar lead from the right subclavian area to V_5 will be adequate in those laboratories which are restricted to testing of subjects with a normal electrocardiogram at rest. In patients with a previous infarction, or other abnormalities in the resting electrocardiogram three (pseudo) orthogonal leads or several standard leads are necessary.
Recommendations for optimal measurements from the exercise electrocardiogram are based on quantitative computer analysis of selected leads in larger groups of patients. Best results were obtained with a combination of ST amplitude, ST slope, and heart rate. The improvement in sensitivity from 50% by visual analysis to 85% by computer was similar to that obtained by body surface mapping. Changes of the P wave and QRS complex during exercise appeared to be of little diagnostic value. The pathophysiological mechanisms which contribute to the changes of the electrocardiogram during exercise are discussed.

Introduction

The first recordings of the electrocradiogram after exercise were made in 1908 by the founder of electrocardiography, Einthoven [1]. Clinical application of post-exercise electrocardiography was induced almost 30 years later, and reviewed by Scherf and Schaffer [2]. In recent years there has been a steady development of exercise electrocardiography towards recording of multiple leads during the whole stress test as well as quantitative analysis of the electrocardiographic changes during and after exercise. However, opinions still differ on basic questions such as lead selection and interpretation of changes of the electrocardiogram during exercise. The answer to these questions may be obtained by quantitative analysis of the whole body surface potential distribution during exercise.
In this paper recommendations are made for the choice of lead systems in various clinical settings, and for the choice of electrocardiographic measurements to be taken during exercise. These recommendations are based on a combination of body surface data in selected patients and quantitative data from selected leads in larger groups of patients. The discussion is restricted to the electrocardiogram. However, it should be understood that other data obtained during an exercise test, such as exercise capacity, heart rate and blood pressure responses and the occurence of chest pain or dyspnea, are of equal value.

---

* Based upon a paper published in The American Journal of Cardiology, Vol. 47 (1981)

Body Surface Potential Distribution at Rest and During Exercise

Body surface maps were recorded with 120 electrodes taped to the chest wall [3]. The recording system has been described in detail [4]. Data were recorded from all leads simultaneously for 8 s with adequate frequency reponse and with a resolution of 20 μV in digital format. After visual inspection of the tracings, beats with similar waveforms were averaged in order to obtain single representative complexes at rest and during exercise with a low noise level. The onset and end of QRS were determined by a computer program and checked by the operator [5]. Exercise was performed on a bicycle ergometer with stepwise workload increments of 25 W each 5 min [3]. Data were recorded at rest, sitting on the bicycle ergometer, at peak exercise and in the first minute of the recovery period.

Body Surface Maps in Normal Subjects

Data were analyzed from 25 normal males, 28–59 years of age. These subjects had no history of cardiovascular disease and were selected on the basis of normal findings in the 12-lead electrocardiogram, chest X-ray, exercise test, and post-exercise thallium scintigraphy [6]. Coronary arteriography was not performed in these subjects. The peak heart rate during exercise averaged 150 beats per minute, range 135–175.

Ventricular depolarization could be characterized by a minimum in the sternal region which shifted gradually toward left lateral and by a minimum at the back or the right shoulder which moved toward the sternum. In most patients a second maximum developed at the end of depolarization in the right subclavian area (Fig. 1).

Repolarization was characterized by a maximum at the mid sternum or at the left sternal border and a minimum which moved from the back towards the anterior part of the right shoulder. These observations were similar to those reported by Taccardi [7] and others [8, 9].

During exercise the depolarization pattern was similar to that at rest (Fig. 2). In 15 out of 25 subjects the amplitudes of the maxima and minima increased by 0.1 mV or more, up to 0.77 mV, while the amplitudes decreased 0.1 mV or more in six subjects (Fig. 3). A reduction of the maximum QRS magnitude was described recently in 20 young subjects [10]. The early repolarization pattern during exercise differed from the pattern at rest. In the first 10–20 ms the potential distribution was similar to the late depolarization patterns. The precordial minimum remained present for 40–100 ms after the end of QRS. The amplitude of this minimum was low: less than 90 μV in all subjects at 60 ms after the end of QRS.

The late repolarization pattern was again similar to the pattern at rest, although the voltages reached the highest values earlier. In 12 subjects the repolarization voltages had the same magnitudes at rest and during exercise, while in eight subjects the voltages during exercise were smaller and in five they were greater.

Mirvis et al. [11] described precordial maps during strenous exercise in 15 normal volunteers. These authors observed similar negative precordial potentials during early repolarization as those described above.

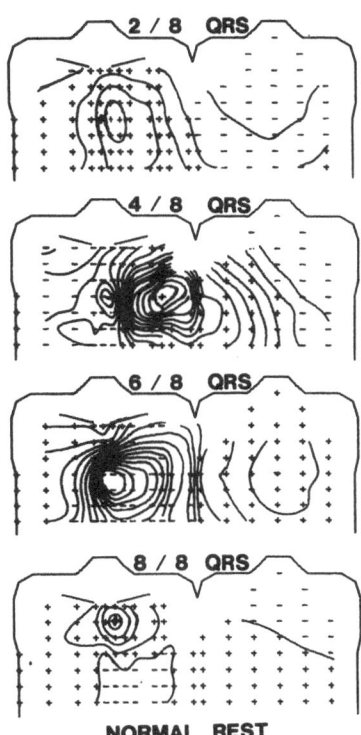

NORMAL REST

Fig. 1. Body surface maps during depolarization in a normal subject at rest. In each diagram the part on the left represents the anterior chest wall while the back is presented in the right. Two lines which represent the clavicles have been drawn in each diagram as well as in the other surface maps. The maps correspond to four time-normalized instants during depolarization at 2/8, 4/8, and 8/8 of QRS duration. Note a maximum in the sternal region during early depolarization (2/8) which shifts towards the left (4/8) and the back (6/8). At the end of depolarization two maxima are present, at the back and at the upper part of the sternum (8/8). The minimum shifts from the back (2/8) through the right side of the chest (4/8), towards the left precordial region (6/8 and 8/8)

Body Surface Maps in Patients with Coronary Artery Disease

Body surface maps were made in 25 male patients with coronary artery disease between 40 and 55 years of age. All had a normal QRS complex and ST segment at rest, and no history of myocardial infarction. Selective coronary arteriography showed 50% or greater luminal narrowing in one or more major coronary arteries. The patients reached an average peak heart rate of 135 beats per minute (range 110–160).

The depolarization maps were similar to the normal maps in 23 patients. Two patients had abnormal negative voltages at the right anterior chest wall during early depolarization. Repolarization at rest was abnormal in five patients, in spite of a normal 12-lead electrocardiogram. These patients had a negative precordial potential which exceeded -50 μV at 60 ms after QRS. During exercise the depolarization potentials increased by 0.1 mV or more in 15 out of 25 patients (Fig. 3), and decreased by this amount in five patients. Thus no systematic difference was observed between the direction or the magnitude of the QRS changes in the normal subjects and in the patients. In six patients an augmentation was observed of the late maximum at the right shoulder or at the right sternal border.

The greatest deviation from the normal pattern was observed in the early repolarization during exercise (Fig. 4). All patients developed a prolonged negative area at the precordium. The precise location of the greatest negative values varied (Fig. 5) [11, 12]. However, no relationship could be observed between the repolarization pattern and the location of

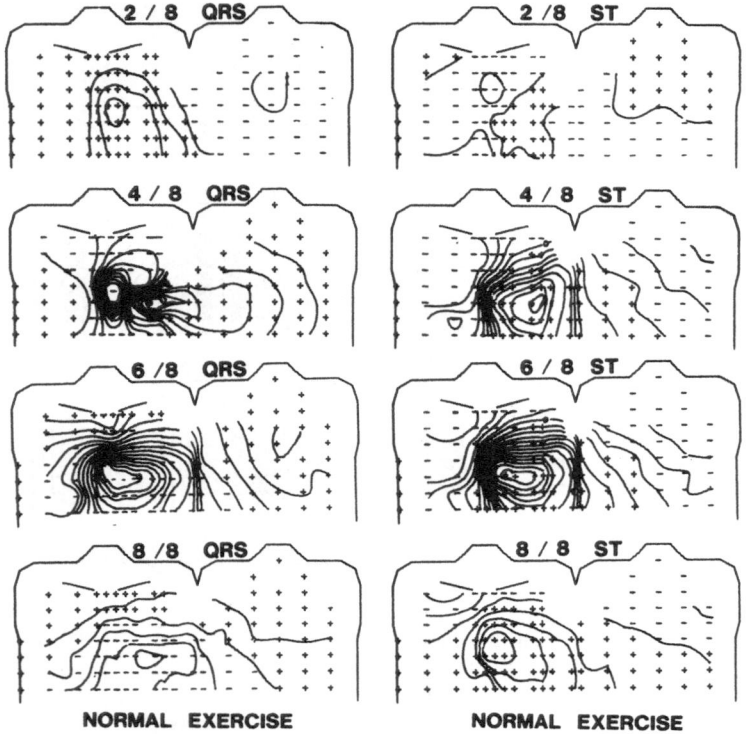

Fig. 2. Normal depolarization pattern during peak exercise. The general pattern is similar to that at rest in the same patient (Fig. 1). During repolarization a maximum develops in the left precordical region (2/8) which remains in the same location but broadens and increases in strength (4/8, 6/8) and diminishes at the end of repolarization

defects in the thallium scintigrams or the location of coronary artery obstructions which confirms earlier reports from our laboratory [13] and others [14].

The Diagnostic Value of Exercise Surface Maps

As might be expected, the surface maps showed abnormal repolarization patterns in some patients with coronary artery disease which were not present in the standard 12-lead electro-cardiogram. A horizontal or down-sloping ST segment depression in the standard chest leads was present in only 15 of the 25 patients. Nevertheless 21 patients had abnormal negative precordial potentials greater than 90 μV at 60 ms after the end of QRS, while such potentials were not present in a single normal subject. The other four patients had a negative precordial area between 50 and 90 μV. Such negative values were also present in three normal subjects (Figs. 5 and 6). The results of this analysis are presented in Table 1.

Similar results have been presented by Fox et al. [12] in a series of 100 patients with 16-lead precordial maps. In their study the sensitivity was 96% with the maps and 80% with the 12-lead system, while the specificity by both methods was the same.

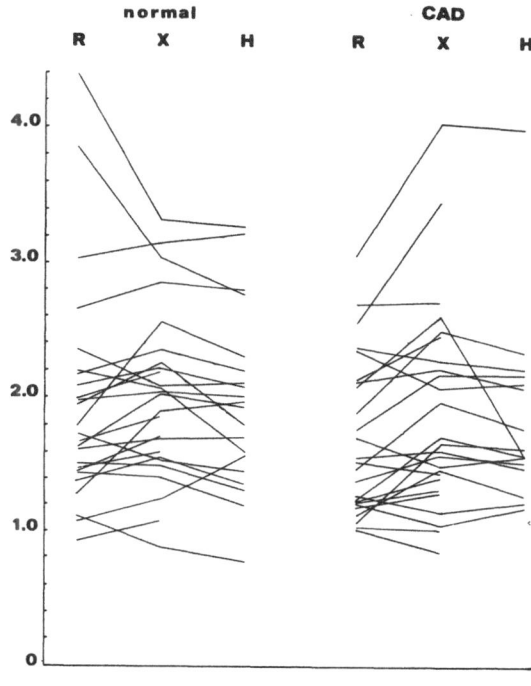

Fig. 3. Maximum QRS amplitudes in the surface maps at rest (R), during peak exercise (X), and in the first minute of recovery (H) in normal subjects *(left)* and in patients with coronary artery disease *(right)*

The presented data were obtained at rest, at peak exercise and in the first minute of the recovery period. Further analysis of the transition of the body surface potential distribution from rest to peak exercise should be performed in order to determine whether abnormal patterns can be detected earlier from the surface maps than from the standard leads.

Table 1. Comparison of sensitivity and specificity in standard precordial leads, in lead X of the Frank orthogonal lead system, in a bipolar chest lead (see text) and in the surface map. ST 60 = ST amplitudes at 60 ms after the end of QRS

	Specificity (n = 25)	Sensitivity (n = 25)
0.1 mV mV horizontal or down-sloping ST ↓ V_2-V_6	100	60
ST 60 $< - 0.045$ mV in X	90	76
ST 60 $< - 0.045$ mV in CS_5	95	84
ST 60 precordial map $< - 0.050$ mV	88	100
ST 60 precordial $< 0,090$ mV	100	84

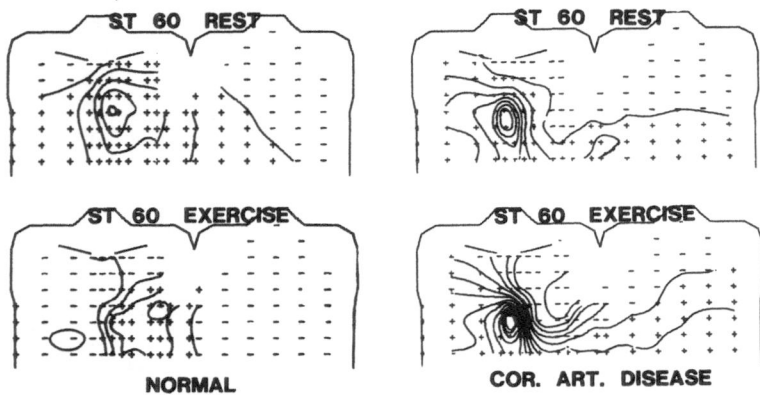

Fig. 4. Body surface maps 60 ms after the end of QRS at rest and at peak exercise in a normal subject (*left*) and in a patient with coronary artery disease. See legend for Fig. 1. Note a broad maximum in the left precordial region in the normal subject, and negative precordial voltages in the patient

The Optimal Lead System for Exercise Electrocardiography

The data in the previous paragraph indicate that the sensitivity of exercise electrocardiography can be increased, without loss of specificity, when a large number of leads are analyzed simultaneously. The optimal lead system will then be a trade-off between a large number of leads and clinical applicability.

The selection of the lead system may be guided by the type of ST patterns which may be expected in a given population. Exercise-induced myocardial ischemia in patients with a normal electrocardiogram at rest is characterized by a negative precordial potential during early repolarization (e.g., ST 60). In such patients the single lead with the highest senstivity will be recorded between the right subclavicular area and the V_5 position (Fig. 4). This is the bipolar lead CS_5 as presented in Table 1. However, in some patients the negative precordial potentials dò not overlap with the V_5 position and multiple leads will be advantageous. This can be extended to a precordial map, such as the 16-lead map (4 x 4) used by Fox et al. [12, 14].

In patients with a previous myocardial infarction the ST changes may be caused by four mechanisms. First, the factors which influence the ST segment in normal subjects should be taken into account, such as heart rate, intracardiac blood volume and the position of the heart in the chest. Secondly, these are modified by the presence of scar tissue or hypokinetic or dyskinetic areas in the left ventricle without ischemia. This will cause largely ST segment elevation in the leads which show the Q waves of the previous infarction [15]. In the third place, myocardial ischemia may be provoked by exercise. In most patients such ischemia occurs in the subendocardial layers of the whole left ventricle. This results in negative precordial potentials, and ST segment depression in the precordial leads. The location of the negative precordial potentials or the orientation of the abnormal ST vectors appears to be independent of the location of the coronary artery obstructions [13, 14, 36]. However, the ST vector orientation will be influenced by the presence of scar tissue due to a previous infarction [15]. Finally, in a few patients, transmural myocardial ischemia may

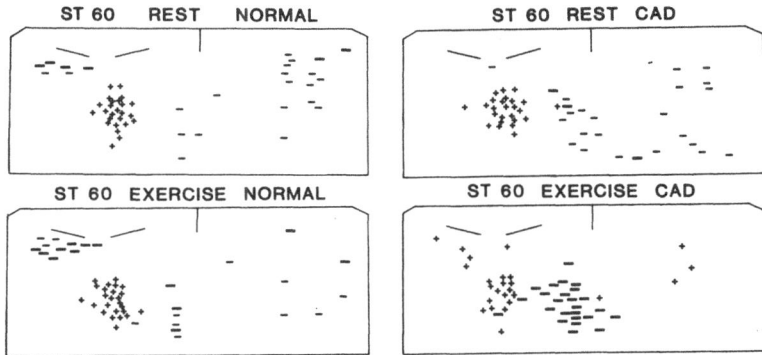

Fig. 5. Distribution of the maxima (+) and the minima (−) of the body surface maps, 60 ms after the end of QRS. See legend Fig. 1. The minima are indicated with a heavy (**−**) sign when the minimal surface potential was lower than −0.050 mV, while a small (−) sign is used for the other subjects. Note maxima in the sternal area both at rest and during exercise in the normal subjects (*left*) and in the patients (*right*). The minima in the normal subjects are located at the back and in the righ subclavian region. In the patients the minima at rest are found at the back and the lower part of the left side of the chest. During exercise the minima are deeper, and all are located in the precordial region

develop, due to coronary spasm. This will result in an area with ST segment elevation over the ischemic zone [16].

In patients with a previous myocardial infarction, it might be of advantage to analyze the whole body surface potential distribution during exercise. A practical approach in research-oriented hospitals would be the reconstruction of the potential distribution from a set of 18–32 leads at specific locations [17, 18]. A further reduction of the number of leads with little loss of information may be obtained through the method described by Kornreich et al. [19]. for the resting electrocardiogram.

Since the repolarization is largely characterized by a single maximum and a single minimum in the surface maps, the representation by a dipole will contain most of the information (Figs. 2 and 4). Thus a corrected orthogonal lead system might be sufficient in all or most patients, provided that precise criteria are developed for spatial analysis of the ST vector. Such criteria have been described for patients with a normal electrocardiogram at rest [20], however data are lacking in patients with a previous myocardial infarction or other abnormalities in the electrocardiogram at rest [15].

In summary, a single bipolar lead (CM_5 or CS_5) will be sufficient in those centers where only subjects with a normal electrocardiogram at rest are tested. In centers with a mixed population, including patients who have had a myocardial infarction, such a system is not sufficient. In those laboratories one should record at least three (pseudo) orthogonal leads [21, 22] in addition to or including CS_5, or a larger set of precordial leads [23, 24]. A corrected orthogonal lead system may be sufficient in the majority of patients, provided that specific criteria are developed which can be used in a computer system.

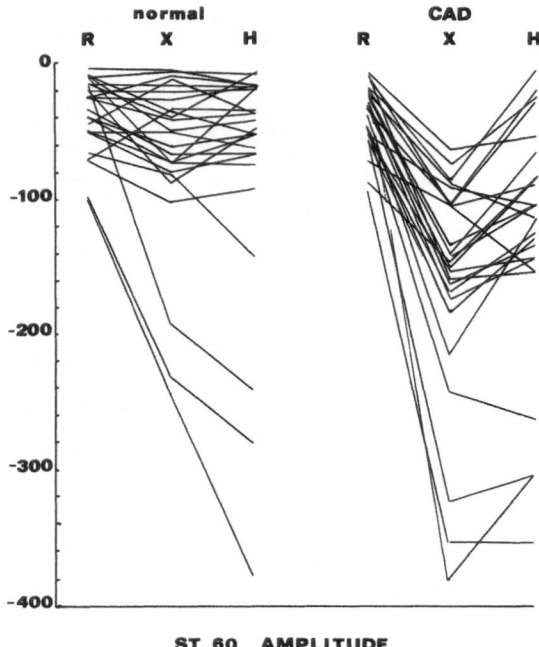

Fig. 6. Amplitudes of the minima of the surface maps at 60 ms after the end of QRS in normal subjects *(left)* and in patients with coronary artery disease *(right)*. See legend Fig. 3

The Most Effective ECG Measurements for Detection of Exercise-Induced Ischemia or Abnormal Myocardial Function

The changes of the P wave, the QRS complex, and the ST-T segement during exercise in patients with coronary artery disease differ from those in normal subjects [15]. In the normals the P wave amplitude increases, the maximum QRS amplitude decreases, the S wave deepens and an ST junction depression occurs [25]. It should be remembered, however, that the changes in individual subjects vary widely, as is illustrated in Fig. 3.

In general, in the patients the P wave amplitudes increase less, the QRS voltages may be enhanced, and both ST depression and ST elevation may occur. For diagnostic use of these changes in the electrocardigram, it should be remembered that in addition to myocardial ischemia or abnormal contraction patterns (when present), the patients generally stop exercise at a lower heart rate than the normal subjects. This factor alone has considerable influence on all measurements from the electrocardiogram [25]. Therefore the most effective measurements should be adjusted for differences in heart rate as has been shown by earlier studies from our laboratory [20].

Differences in P waves between patients and normal subjects during exercise have little diagnostic value if any (Table 2). These differences are probably largely due to the lower peak heart rate in the patients, although they may be affected by elevated left ventricular filling pressure in some patients [26, 27].

The surface map data indicate that the precordial QRS potentials in most patients increase during exercise, as well as those in the normal subjects. No systematic difference was observed between magnitude of these changes in the two groups (Fig. 3). This is at variance with recent reports that augmentation of the R waves during exercise can be used as an indication

Table 2. Sensitivity of P, QRS, and ST measurements for detection of coronary artery disease in male patients with a normal ECG at rest (n = 53). Measurements at the highest exercise level in each patient. Threshold values were selected such that the specificity was approximately 90% in 87 normal subjects

Parameter		Sensitivity		Specificity	
P max	X	14/53	(.26)	76/87	(.88)
	Y	15/53	(.28)	78/87	(.90)
	Z	1/53	(.01)	78/87	(.90)
QRS 6/8	X	13/53	(.24)	78/87	(.90)
	Y	9/53	(.16)	78/87	(.90)
	Z	6/53	(.11)	78/87	(.90)
QRS 7/8	X	12/53	(.22)	78/87	(.90)
	Y	10/53	(.18)	78/87	(.90)
	Z	8/53	(.15)	78/87	(.90)
ST 4/8	X	35/53	(.66)	77/87	(.89)
	Y	23/53	(.43)	78/87	(.90)
	Z	2/53	(.03)	78/87	(.90)
ST 60	X	53/53	(.66)	78/87	(.90)
	Y	23/53	(.43)	78/87	(.90)
	Z	0/53	(.00)	78/87	(.90)

of the presence of coronary artery disease [28]. It should be noted that R waves changes in that study [28] were analyzed in a single lead only. Thus the observed differences in R wave changes could be due to minor shifts in the location of the maximum QRS potentials at the chest wall (Figs. 1 and 2).

Furthermore, the R wave changes are related to heart rate. At submaximal workloads, R wave amplitudes increase in normal subjects, while decreased amplitudes occur at high heart rates [30]. The differences between R wave changes in normals and in patients may therefore be due also in part to the lower peak heart rates in the latter group.

Finally, it has been suggested that the larger R wave changes which have been observed in coronary artery disease are caused by enlarged left ventricular volumes due to myocardial dysfunction [28]. However, experimental data to support this mechanism are lacking. One study even reported no relation between R wave changes and left ventricular volumes measured by bloodpool scintigraphy [29]. Data from our laboratory indicate that the R wave changes are dependent, like the ST changes, on the presence and the location of a previous myocardial infarction (Table 3). Thus more experimental and clinical data are required to define the significance of differences in QRS measurements between various groups of patients [31].

A wealth of information is available on the ST segment changes during exercise. Both a horizontal or down-sloping ST segment depression and a slowly ascending ST segment have been associated with coronary artery disease [32]. The likelihood of an abnormal (ischemic) ST segment response is greater when the ST segment depression (1) is of greater magnitude, measured at the J point or up to 80 ms after QRS; (2) has a more horizontal or negative slope; (3) occurs at a lower heart rate, or earlier during the test; and (4) is associated with other symptoms such as chest pain and a lack of rise or drop of systolic blood pressure.

Table 3. Sensitivities of the changes between rest and highest exercise level in 53 patients with coronary artery disease and a normal ECG at rest (CAD); in 49 patients with a previous anteroseptal (AMI) and in 61 patients with a previous inferior, or posterior wall infarction (PMI). The parameters with the highest sensitivities in each group have been included. Threshold levels were selected such that the specificity was 90% in a group of 87 normal subjects

Parameter			CAD		AMI		PMI	
P max		X	19/53	(.35)	19/49	(.38)	26/61	(.42)
QRS	6/8	X	19/53	(.35)	28/49	(.57)	22/61	(.16)
	7/8	Y	6/53	(.11)	5/59	(.10)	22/61	(.36)
	7/8	Z	18/53	(.33)	4/49	(.08)	23/61	(.37)
ST	70	X	34/53	(.64)	9/49	(.18)	29/61	(.47)
	90	Y	37/53	(.69)	11/49	(.22)	28/61	(.45)
	70	Z	11/53	(.20)	4/49	(.08)	19/61	(.31)
ST	4/8	X	7/53	(.13)	7/49	(.14)	30/61	(.49)
	5/8	Y	23/53	(.43)	3/49	(.06)	23/61	(.37)
	5/8	Z	8/53	(.15)	25/49	(.51)	3/61	(.04)

Several studies have shown that the diagnostic value of exercise electrocardiography can be enhanced by computer processing, both for enhancement of the signal-noise ratio and for application of specific measurements. Comparison of a large number of measurements has shown that the highest diagnostic performance is obtained by combination of ST amplitudes and ST slopes measured at fixed intervals after QRS in the first 100 ms of the ST segment. Such measurements were superior to ST time integrals, time-normalized ST amplitudes and polynomial fits of the ST segment [20, 33–36]. The optimal points where measurements should be taken are dependent on the algorithms for definition of the onset and end of QRS [36, 37]. The data in Fig. 7 indicate that the best single measurement was the ST amplitude 60 ms after the end of QRS, and that a further improvement could be obtained by combination of ST amplitude with heart rate and with ST slope.

Through visual reading of the exercise electrocardiogram, changes of the ST segment can be measured in steps of 0.1 mV (1 mm). Therefore, in clinical practice the same criteria are applied to various leads. When more accurate measurements are taken with the aid of a computer system, specific criteria should be developed for each different lead, or combination of leads.

Such quantitative data provide the additional advantage that the changes in the electrocariogram can be expressed as a probability figure indicating the degree of normality or abnormality [35, 38]. This seems a more logical approach than a yes or no statement, based on arbitrary threshold values for the ST segment measurements.

Discussion

In the preceeding paragraphs, two different approaches have been described towards optimal exercise electrocardiography.

The first approach is the analysis of a large number of electrocardiographic leads. Whole body surface potential distributions during and after exercise have been studied in small

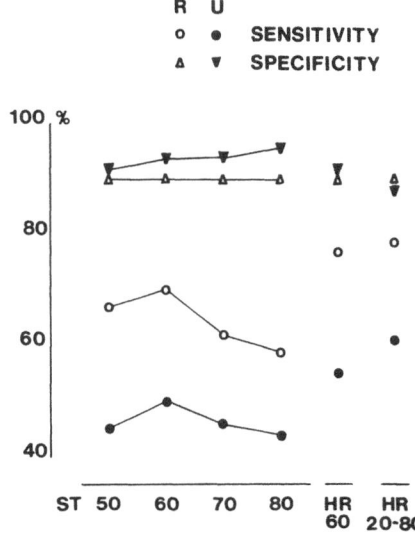

Fig. 7. Comparison of the sensitivity and specificity of various ST amplitudes in two groups of subjects studied at the Thoraxcenter in Rotterdam (R) and at the St. Antonius Hospital in Utrecht (U), The Netherlands. See [36]. The selection of the patients in the two series was different. In Rotterdam 73 patients with coronary artery disease were compared with 125 healthy volunteers without coronary arteriography. In Utrecht the population consisted of 51 "normal" patients with chest pain but without significant lesions at coronary arteriography, and of 96 patients with coronary artery disease. All subjects had a normal 12-lead electrocardiogram at rest. In addition, the Utrecht subjects had a normal exercise test at a previous occasion. This explains the lower sensitivity obtained in Utrecht for the same criteria [36]. Visual reading of the electrocardiograms yielded sensitivities of 50% and 25% and specificities of 95% and 100% in the Rotterdam and Utrecht population respectively. Thresholds for the various computer measurements were selected such that the specificity was 90% in the 125 normal subjects from Rotterdam. Note that the best single measurement in both populations was the ST amplitude 60 ms after the end of QRS. A further improvement could be obtained by combination of the ST amplitude with heart rate (HR 60) and by combination of two ST amplitudes, or ST amplitude and slope, with heart rate (HR 20–80)

series of patients. Larger series have been reported by Fox et al. [12, 14] who recorded 16 precordial leads in 4 x 4 array. A visual reading of these electrocardiograms yielded improved diagnostic value in comparison with standard 12 leads. Such a lead system can easily be applied; however, it does not represent the whole body surface potential distribution.

The second approach requires a more detailed computer analysis of a few leads. With such analysis a similar diagnostic improvement has been reported as with the 16-lead precordial map.

The next step should be a combination of both approaches. This requires recording of precordial and whole body surface potential maps both during and after exercise in large series of patients. For each lead position the normal range of measurements from the QRS complex and the ST segment should be defined. These normal ranges will probably be related to sex, age, body dimensions, and heart rate during exercise and possibly to the type of test protocol which is used. From such material the optimal combination of leads and criteria can be defined.

It is possible that further studies will provide better criteria for exercise electrocardiography than those which have been presented above. However, the additional gain will be limited since both precordial mapping and computer analysis already yield sensitivities between 80% and 90% at a specificity of 90%–95% [12, 20, 35]. This improvement of sensitivity of the exercise electrocardiogram by computer processing or by precordial mapping is of the same magnitude as the improvement obtained by nuclear imaging techniques [39–41].

At the end of this paper it seems appropriate to remind the reader that even the most sophisticated analysis of the exercise electrocardiogram cannot replace clinical judgement based on a combination of all data available on a given patient. This should include a careful history, determination of exercise tolerance and the hemodynamic response to exercise, as well as, in some patients, analysis of wall motion and global ventricular function from blood-pool scintigrams [39] and an estimation of myocardial perfusion patterns and cellular function from thallium scintigraphy [41].

Acknowledgements. The data in Fig. 7 have been collected and analyzed as part of a cooperative study of the St. Antonius Hospital in Utrecht, the Thoraxcenter of the Erasmus University in Rotterdam and Unit for Cardiovascular Research of the Free University in Brussels.

References

1 Einthoven W (1908) Weiteres über das Elektrokardiogram. Arch Ges Physiol Menschen Thiere 122:517–520
2 Scherf D, Schaffer AI (1952) The electrocardiographic exercise test. Am Heart J 43: 927–946
3 Block P, Lenaers A, Tiberghien J et al (1976) Surface maps and myocardial scanning at rest and during exercise: Comparison with coronary angiography. Acta Cardiol (Brux) 31:467–481
4 Tiberghien J, Steenhaut O, Lenders P, Block P, Kornreich F (1976) An 128-channel electrocardiographic recorder. Adv Cardiol 16:128–132
5 Block P, Tiberghien J, Raadschelder I, Coussaert E, Lenaers A, Bourgain R, Kornreich F (1978) Diagnostic value of surface mapping recordings registered at rest and during exercise. Comp Cardiol 89–93
6 Lenaers A, Block P, van Thiel E, Lebedelle M et al (1977) Segmental analysis of Tl-201 stress myocardial scintigraphy. J Nucl Med 18:509–516
7 Taccardi B (1963) Distribution of heart potentials in the thoracic surface of normal human subjects. Circ Res 12:341–352
8 Horan L, Flowers N, Brody O (1963) Body surface potential distribution. Circ Res 13: 373–387
9 Spach MS, Barr RC, Blumenschein SD, Boineau JP (1968) Clinical implications of iso-potential surface maps. Ann Intern Med 69:919–928
10 Miller WT, Spach MS, Warren RB (1980) Total body surface potential mapping during exercise: QRS-T wave changes in normal young adults. Circulation 62 3:632)645
11 Mirvis DM, Keller FW Jr, Cox JW, Zettergen DG, Dowdie RF, Ideker RE (1979) Left precordial isopotential mapping during supine exercise. Circulation 56:245–252
12 Fox KM, Selwyn A, Shillingford JP (1979) Precordial electrographic mapping after exercise in the diagnosis of coronary artery disease. Am J Cardiol 43:541–546

13 Simoons ML, Withagen A, Vinke R, Kooy P, Bakker W (1978) ST-Vector orientation and location of myocardial perfusion defects during exercise. Nucl Med 17 4:154—156

14 Fox KM, Selwyn A, Oakley D, Shillingford JP (1979) Relation between the procordial projection of ST segment changes after exercise and coronary angiographic findings. Am J Cardiol 44:1068—1075

15 Simoons ML, van den Brand M, Hugenholtz PG (1977) Quantitative analysis of exercise electrocardiograms and left ventricular angiograms in patients with abnormal QRS complexes at rest. Circulation 55:55—60

16 Waters DD, Chaitman BR, Bourassa MG, Tubau JF (1980) Clinical and angiographic correlates of exercise-induced ST-segment elevation. Circulation 61:286—296

17 Warren RB, Barr RC, Spach MS (1977) Determining the minimum number and best placement of leads for a practical clinical body surface mapping system (abstract) Circulation 56 III:200

18 Yanowitz FG, Vincent GM, Lux RL, Merchant M, Davis D (1980) Clinical applications of body surface ECG mapping during exercise testing. In: Proceedings of 1980 Engineering Foundation Conference "Computerized Interpretation of the ECG V". pp 1—8

19 Kornreich F (1973) The missing waveform information in the orthogonal electrocardiogram (Frank leads). I. Where and how can this missing waveform information be trieved. Circulation 48:984—995

20 Simoons ML (1977) Optimal measurements for detection of coronary artery disease by exercise echocardiography. Comput Biomed Res 10:483—499

21 Froehlicher VF, Thompson AJ, Longo MR, Triebwasser JH, Lancaster MC (1976) Value of exercise testing for screening asymptomatic men for latent coronary artery disease. Prog Cardiovasc Dis 18 4:265—276

22 Ellestad MH (1975) Stress testing: Principles and practice. Davis, Philadelphia

23 Tubau JF, Chaitman BR, Bourassa MG, Waters DD (1980) Detection of multivessel coronary disease after myocardial infarction using exercise stress testing and multiple ECG lead systems. Circulation 61:44—52

24 Berman JL, Wynne J, Cohn PF (1980) Multiple lead QRS changes with exercise testing. Circulation 61:53—61

25 Simoons ML, Hugenholtz PG (1975) Gradual changes of ECG waveform during and after exercise in normal subjects. Circulation 52:570—577

26 Roskam H, Samek L, Rupp G, Schnellbacher K, Petersen J, Stürzen-Hofecker P, Rentrop P, Prokoph J (1977) Verbessert die zusätzliche Messung des Pulmonalkapillardruckes während körperlicher Belastung die Voraussage des koronarangiographischen Befundes bei Patienten ohne transmuralen Herzinfarkt? Z Kardiol 66:477—482

27 Heikkilä J, Hugenholtz PG, Tabakin BS (1973) Prediction of left heart filling pressure and its sequential change in acute myocardial infarction from the terminal force of the P wave. Br Heart J 35:142—151

28 Bonoris PE, Greenberg PS, Castellanet MJ, Ellestad MH (1978) Significance of changes in R-wave amplitude during treadmill stress testing: Angiographic correlation. Am J Cardiol 41:846—851

29 Wolthuis RA, Froelicher VF, Hopkirk A, Fischer JR, Keiser N (1979) Normale electrocardiographic waveform characteristics during treadmill exercise testing. Circulation 60:1028—1035

30 Battler A, Froehlicher V, Slutsky R, Ashburn W (1979) Relationship of QRS amplitude changes during exercise to left ventricular function and volumes and the diagnosis of coronary artery disease. Circulation 60 5:1004—1013

31 Simoons ML (1979) QRS changes in CAD (Letter to the editor) Circulation 59 4:841—843

32 Rijneke RD, Ascoop CA, Talmon JL (1980) Clinical significance of upsloping ST segments in exercise electrocardiography. Circulation 61:671—678

33 Ascoop CA, Distelbrink CA, de Lang PA, van Bemmel JH (1974) Quantitaitve comparison of exercise vectorcardiograms and findings at selective coronary arteriography. J Electrocardiol 7:9—16

34   Ascoop CA, Distelbrink CA, de Lang PA (1977) Clinical value of quantitative analysis of ST slop during exercise. Br Heart J 39:212)217

35   Hollenberg M, Budge WR, Wisneski JA, Gertz EW (1980) Treadmill score-qualifies electrocardiographic response to exercise and improves test accuracy and reproducibility. Circulation 61:276–285

36   Simoons ML, Ascoop CA, Distelbrink CA, Block P, de Lang P, Vinke R (1977) Computer processing of exercise electrocardiograms. In: James WE, Amsterdam E (eds) Coronary heart disease, exercise testing and cardiac rehabilitation. Symposia Specialists, Miami, pp 155–164

37   Simoons ML, Hugenholtz PG, Ascoop CA, Distelbrink CA, de Lang PA, Vinke R (1981) Quantitation of exercise electrocardiography. Circulation 63:471–476

38   Simoons ML, Hugenholtz PG (1979) Estimation of the probability of exercise induced ischemia by quantitative ECG analysis. Circulation 56:552–559

39   Bodenheimer MM, Banka VS, Helfant RH (1980) Review on radionuclide angiographic assessment of left ventricular contraction: Uses, limitations and future directions. Am J Cardiol 45:661–673

40   Bodenheimer MM, Banka VS, Helfant RH (1980) Review on the role of myocardial perfusion imaging using thallium-201 in diagnosis of coronary heart disease. Am J Cardiol 45:674–684

41   Okada RD, Boucher CA, Strauss HW, Pohost GM (1980) Exercise radionuclide imaging approaches to coronary artery disease. Am J Cardiol 46:1188–1204

Coronary Angiography

P. Mathes

The need for any diagnostic test must be evaluated on the basis of the information it provides, the risk of the test, whether the same information could be provided by another, possibly less risky and less costly test, and the therapy it leads to. At present, coronary angiography is the only test that provides information about the site, extent, and severity of obstructive coronary artery disease. However, several questions about this procedure still remain unanswered. The ad hoc committee of the American Heart Association recommended in 1977 that *routine* coronary artery angiography after acute myocardial infarction was not indicated. There are, however, several authors who assert that there is a need for routine coronary angiography after acute myocardial infarction. The following reasons are given most frequently:

1. *To assess prognosis:* Angiographic studies have shown that the severity of coronary artery obstruction and the degree of left ventricular dysfunction are two major factors which influence survival in patients with coronary artery disease [1, 5, 6, 9, 10].
   Angiographic studies of survivors of myocardial infarction have suggested a high incidence of multivessel coronary artery disease. From recent studies [2, 20] we have learned that the clinical course of patients with coronary artery disease is quite variable, even within the usual categories of one, two, and three-vessel disease or main stem stenosis. Still, in three-vessel disease only 50% of patients are alive at the end of 10 years, in contrast to the 10%–20% mortality of patients with single-vessel disease. Consequently, coronary angiography is of help in assessing prognosis in the individual patient, and the need to assess prognosis can be regarded as a valid reason for recommending coronary angiography in certain patients following myocardial infarction.

2. *To recommend a program of physical exercise following myocardial infarction:* The limits of exercise tolerance can be safely defined by noninvasive stress testing such as bicycle-ergometry and by radionuclide studies determining ventricular function under exercise. Thus, for the sole purpose of determining the safe margins of an exercise program, coronary angiography is not required. However, exercise studies following myocardial infarction are of limited value in detecting myocardium jeopardized by ischemia, and this limited sensitivity precludes their use as the yardstick for the final decision about the future management of the patient, particularly in the younger age group.

3. *To determine optimal medical management:* In regard to optimal medical management, it is not clear how knowledge of the site and extent of coronary artery obstruction would influence the decision about medical treatment. In the symptomatic patient following myocardial infarction, treatment will be given in accordance with the symptoms presented. In trials of secondary prevention after myocardial infarction, the routine administration of β-blocking agents has so far shown beneficial effects [9, 10, 12, 18, 20]. In these studies, coronary angiography was not required as an entry criterion; consequently, if treatment is given on this basis, coronary angiography will not be required.

4. *To determine optimal surgical therapy:* There is currently little doubt that surgery prolongs life in patients with left main stem and three-vessel coronary disease. In certain

subsets of patients with doube- and single-vessel disease, successful bypass surgery improves prognosis as well. It needs to be emphasized, however, that benefit obtained from coronary artery bypass surgery is prolonging the life of patients with coronary disease has been proven only in symptomatic patients [3, 4, 11]. Clearly, at a given stage of coronary artery disease the question of symptoms will largely depend upon the level of physical and emotional activity. Personality traits and denial will also influence the degree to which the symptoms are presented. One can therefore cautiously conclude that it appears reasonable to extrapolate the results observed in symptomatic patients to those patients presenting without severe symptoms, although data to substantiate this statement are still lacking.

A crucial point is the sensitivity of nonivasive procedures in determining the extent of coronary disease in patients following myocardial infarction. One of the questions concerns the appropriate time to perform such studies. In the patient immediately recovering from acute myocardial infarction, loss of exercise capability is partly due to deconditioning of peripheral musculature, and thus may lead to an early cessation of exercise tests. Consequently, the yield of such exercise tests may be low.

In our series of 500 consecutive patients undergoing selective coronary angiography, left main stem disease was present to a significant degree in 4.5%. In all of these patients, evidence of exercise-induced ischemia in the surviving myocardium was suggested either by the presence of angina pectoris on effort, by an ischemic response in the exercise ECG, or by the occurrence of an additional perfusion defect in the thallium-201 image on exercise. Thus, in our experience, the patient with significant left main stem disease following myocardial infarction who is asymptomatic is extremely rare; in fact, following an adequately controlled reconditioning program, it could be stated that either subjective or objective evidence of myocardial ischemia below the submaximal exercise level is present in all patients with significant left main coronary artery obstruction.

The relationship between the extent of coronary artery disease and the occurrence of angina pectoris and stress-inducible myocardial ischemia is less strict in three-vessel disease. In a recent report [17], exercise stress testing, electrocardiographic location of the infarction, total sum cholesterol, and clinical features, including blood pressure, smoking habits, family history of coronary artery disease, and the presence of angina pectoris either before of after the acute event, proved to be poor predictors of multiple-vessel disease in patients below the age of 45. In our own series of 500 patients undergoing coronary angiography, the predictive accuracy of exercise stress testing in three-vessel disease did not reach the same degree as in left main coronary artery disease. Particularly in men below the age of 45, all three major vessels may be obstructed without severe symptoms, even in the presence of a normal exercise tolerance test. It therefore appears possible to recommend coronary angiography in this particular group of patients after myocardial infarction, even in the absence of symptoms.

In conclusion, it is currently not possible to recommend *routine* coronary angiography for *all* patients following acute myocardial infarction. There is a certain subset of patients with severe coronary disease who will benefit from coronary artery surgery, not only in regard to their symptoms but also in regard to their prognosis. Particularly in patients below 45 years, it is difficult to identify this group by nonivasive techniques. In the older age group, the patient with multiple-vessel disease can be more easily identified by the presence of anginal symptoms, an abnormal exercise ECG, or an exercise-induced perfusion defect in thallium imaging in the remaining myocardium after myocardial infarction. The patient who, following myocardial infarction, is entirely free of anginal symptoms and, after an appropriate training period, is able to perform an exercise test reaching the submaximal heart rate without subjective or objective signs of myocardial ischemia, and yet still presents with a severe degree of coronary obstruction in the left main coronary artery, appears to be an extremely rare exception. In order to intelligently advise a program of physical exercise and to define the optimal medical management, prior coronary angiography is not necessarily required. However, significant obstruction of the three major coronary vessels may be present in patients following myocardial infarction, particularly in the age group below 45 years, without clinical signs of angina or ischemia provoked by stress testing. Aside from this particular group, it appears reasonable to restrict coronary angiography to those patients who, following myocardial infarction, demonstrate ischemia in the residual, surviving myocardium either subjectively by angina pectoris or objectively by signs of myocardial ischemia on exercise stress testing.

References

1 Burggraf GW, Parker JO (1975) Prognosis in coronary artery disease. Angiographic, hemodynamic and clinical factors. Circulation 51:146

2 Corne RA, Gotsman MS, Weiss A et al (1979) Thallium-201 scintigraphy in diagnosis of coronary stenosis. Comparison with electrocardiography and coronary arteriography. Br Heart J 41:575–583

3 DeMots H, Bonchek LI, Rösch J et al (1975) Left main coronary artery disease: risks of angiography, importance of coexisting disease of other coronary arteries and effects or revascularization. Am J Cardiol 36:136–141

4 DeMots H, Rösch J, McAnulty JH et al (1977) Left main coronary artery disease. In: Rahimtoola SH (ed) Coronary bypass surgery. FA Davis, Philadelphia, pp 201–212

5 Friesinger GC, Page EF, Ross RS (1970) Prognostic significance or coronary arteriography. Trans Assoc Am Physicians 83:78–92

6 Humphries JO, Kuller L, Ross RS et al (1974) Natural history of ischemic heart disease in relation to arteriographic findings. Circulation 49:489–497

7 Hurst JW, Logue RB, Walter PF (1978) Recognition and management of coronary atherosclerotic heart disease. In: Hurst JW, Logue RB, Schlant RC, Wenger NK (eds) The heart. McGraw-Hill, New York, p 1260

8 Madigan NP, Rutherford BD, Frye RL (1976) The clinical course, early prognosis and coronary anatomy of subendocardial infarction. Am J Med 60:634–641

9 Multicentre International Study (1975) Improvement in prognosis of myocardial infarction by long-term beta-adrenoreceptor blockade using practolol: a multicentre international study. Br Med J III:735–740

10 Multicentre International Study (1977) Reduction in mortality with long-term beta-adrenoceptor blockade: a multicentre international study. Br Med J II:49–51

11 Norris RM, Agnew TM, Brandt PWT et al (1981) Coronary surgery after recurrent myocardial infarction: progress of a trial comparing surgical with nonsurgical management for asymptomatic patients with advances coronary disease. Circulation 63:785–792

12 Norwegian Multicenter Study Group (1981) Timolol-induced reduction in mortality and reinfarction in patients surviving acute myocardial infarction. N Engl J Med 304:801–807

13 Oberman A, Jones WB, Riley CP et al (1972) Natural history of coronary artery disease. Bull NY Acad Med 48:1109–1125

14 Rahimtoola SH (1977) Coronary arteriography in asymptomatic patients after myocardial infarction. Chest 77:53–57

15 Reeves TJ, Oberman A, Jones WB et al (1974) Natural history of angina pectoris. Am J Cardiol 33:423−430

16 Schultz RA Jr, Pitt B, Griffith LSC et al (1978) Coronary angiography and left ventriculography in survivors of transmural and nontransmural myocardial infarction. Am J Med 64:108−113

17 Schultz RA Jr, Humphries JO, Griffith LSC et al (1977) Left ventricular and coronary angiographic anatomy. Relationship to ventricular irritability in the late hospital phase of acute myocardial infarction. Circulation 55:839−843

18 Steinbrunn W, Lichtlen P (1977) Complete 5 year cumulative survival rates in 244 unselected, unoperatied coronary patients undergoing angiography. Circulation 55/56: III−174

19 Vanhaecke J, Piessens J, Willems JL, De Gest H (1981) Coronary arterial lesions in young men who survived a first myocardial infarction: Clinical and electrocardiographic predictors of multivessel disease. Am J Cardiol 47:810−814

20 Vedin A, Wilhelmsson C, Elmfeldt D, Säve-Söderberg J, Tibblin G, Wilhelmsen L (1975) Death and non-fatal reinfarction during two years' follow-up after myocardial infarction: a follow-up study of 440 men and women discharged alive from hospital. Acta Med Scand 198:353−364

21 Wilhelmsson C, Vedin JA, Wilhelmsen L, Tibblin G, Werkö L (1974) Reduction of sudden death after myocardial infarction by treatment with alprenolol: preliminary results. Lancet II:865−868

Ambulatory Electrocardiographic Monitoring

K.-P. Bethge and P.R. Lichtlen

Introduction

The interest in long-term electrocardiographic monitoring is still increasing in view of the fact that ventricular dysrhythmias are the major etiologic factor determining sudden coronary death.

A typical example is a 68-year-old male patient 16 years after anterior myocardial infarction demonstrating episodes of ventricular tachycardia during ambulatory monitoring (Fig. 1) despite a history free of palpitations. Undoubtedly, during the period of ventricular tachycardia the patient is at increased risk of sudden cardiac death. This is further stressed by the syncopes the patient had experienced before admission to hospital, which initially were assumed to be neurologic.

Since several groups could demonstrate increased ectopic activity in victims of sudden death and the occurrence of complex forms, respectively, preceding the fatal outcome [11, 18, 19, 24, 25, 28], the question arises: Which technique is able to reliably detect spontaneous dysrhythmias indicating electrical instability of the heart?

Diagnostic Sensitivity of the Routine-ECG, Exercise Stress Testing and Long-Term ECG-Monitoring

The most commonly used electrocardiographic methods in clinical cardiology are the 12-lead ECG at rest ("routine ECG"), exercise stress testing and long-term monitoring of the ECG. We compared the incidence of uniform and complex ventricular extrasystoles (multiform VES, bigeminal rhythm and/or consecutive VES) in 93 patients (88 men and five women; age: 32–65 years, mean age 50 years) with documented coronary artery disease, using all three methods (Fig. 2).

Every medication was withdrawn at least 2 days prior to the test with the exception of digitalis and/or nitrates in patients with congestive heart failure and/or severe angina.

The time spent exercising the patients in the supine position on a bicycle was 9 min, with a recovery period of an additional 6 min. Age- and sex-dependent workloads at three levels, with a duration of 3 min each, were set in accordance with Bühlmann's proposal [7]. Rhythm analysis during and after stress testing was obtained by continuous monitoring of six chest wall leads (V_{1-6}) (Fa. Siemens, Erlangen, Germany) and a six channel tracing (Cardirex 62, Siemens-Elema, Erlangen, Germany) recorded at 50 mm/s every minute. With increasing ectopic activity continuous ECG recordings at 10 mm/s were performed.

Twenty-four-hour ambulatory monitoring of the ECG was performed using a dual channel tape recorder (Oxford Medilog 4–24, Abingdon, England) with a frequency response of 0.15–100 Hz. Analysis of the tapes was performed at high speed (60:1) with a computer-aided scanning system (Pathfinder II, Reynolds Medical, Hertfort, England) completed by means of a CBS module (Fa. Emetron, Unterhaching, Germany) recently described [32]. Despite

♂ G.W. 68 years old   LZ-EKG 59/80

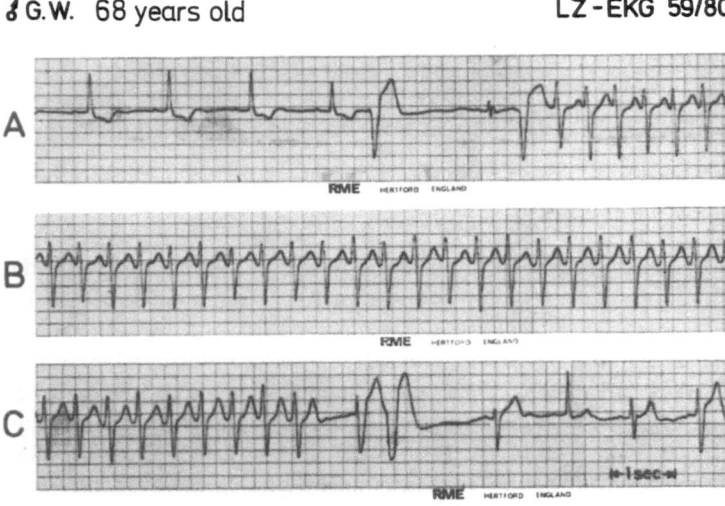

VWI 1964, Rezidiv. VT   260280 C

Fig. 1. Continuous recording (A → B → C) of an episode of ventricular tachycardia from ambulatory ECG monitoring in a 68-year-old male patient 16 years after anterior myocardial infarction

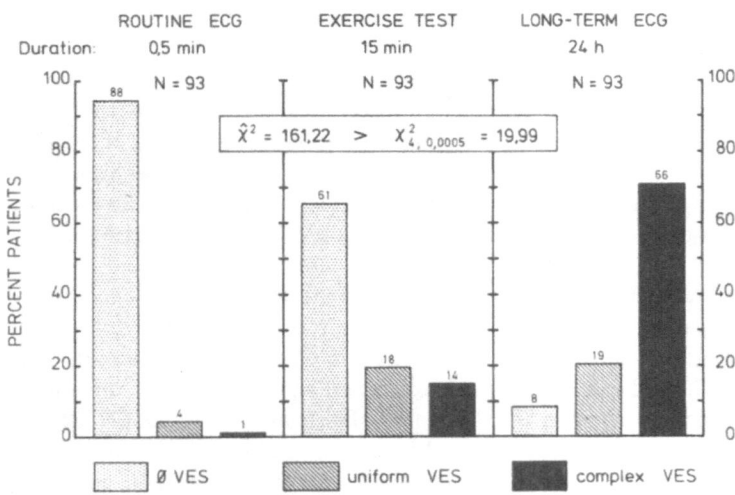

Fig. 2. Comparison of routine ECG, exercise stress testing and ambulatory ECG monitoring in detecting ventricular extrasystoles (VES) in 93 chronic coronary patients. The *numbers above the bars* indicate the number of patients whereas the *height of the bars* indicate the percentage of patients. $\hat{\chi}^2 = 161.22$ = test statistics including all numbers of patients. χ^2_4; 0.0005 = 19.99 = tabulated chi-square referring to a degree of freedom of 4 and a level of significance of 0.05%

high sensitivity and specificity of the hybrid computer (both > 90%) [17] we validated multiform ectopics and bigeminal rhythm as well as all repetitive forms of ventricular extrasystoles by visual analysis from ECG recordings at 25 mm/s.

Figure 2 shows the incidence of uniform and complex ectopics obtained with each method. Only five patients showed ectopics using the 12-lead ECG at rest in contrast to 32 patients (34%) undergoing exercise stress testing. With long-term ECG monitoring even 85 of the 93 coronary patients (91%) revealed ventricular ectopic activity. Complex dysrhythmias such as multiform ectopics, bigeminal rhythm and/or repetitive forms were detected only in a single patient with the routine ECG, in 14 patients (15%) with stress testing, and in 66 patients (71%) using ambulatory ECG monitoring. Thus, multifield-χ^2-analysis confirms significant differences between the three methods ($P < 0.0005$) suggesting high sensitivity of ambulatory monitoring in detecting ventricular ectopy (Fig. 2).

A more detailed comparison between stress testing and ambulatory ECG monitoring (Table 1) demonstrates that only a single patient showed complex ventricular extrasystoles with exercise, but no ectopics with long-term ECG monitoring and another three patients revealed complex ectopics while being exercised but only uniform ectopics during ambulatory monitoring following normal daily activities. Consistent findings of both methods were documented in 19 patients. In contrast to these figures, 54 patients demonstrated uniform and/or complex ventricular extrasystoles with ambulatory ECG monitoring only, these being not detectable with stress testing. Furthermore, another 16 patients demonstrated uniform ventricular extrasystoles while undergoing stress testing, but showed complex forms of ectopic activity with long-term ECG monitoring. In conclusion, ambulatory ECG monitoring is not only the more sensitive method for detecting dysrhythmias but also provides more complete information in most instances, since exercise stress testing adds further information only in a small percentage of patients.

Similar findings from other laboratories have been published in recent years [10, 12, 15, 29, 31, 33].

The basic difference between this study and preceding investigations consists of the use of a hybrid computer [26, 27] in the analysis of 24-h tapes, thus achieving a more marked sensitivity of ambulatory ECG monitoring in detecting transient dysrhythmias.

Duration of Ambulatory ECG-Monitoring

The diagnostic sensitivity of ambulatory ECG monitoring is mainly due to the duration of the monitoring period (Fig. 1) [14]. Since 24-h monitoring includes complete day and night periods this has become the standard time base. Due to the marked spontaneous variability of VES [1, 2, 21, 23, 34] sensitivity decreases with shorter monitoring periods [14] and it becomes more difficult to assess the efficacy of antiarrhythmic therapy. With longer monitoring periods, however, workload of tape analysis increases disproportionately to additional information.

With a new approach of discontinuous ambulatory ECG monitoring, longer storage periods are possible depending on the frequency of dysrhythmias detected. But their spontaneous variability causes a shifting time base from tape to tape even in the same patient, thereby adding further difficulties to the judgement of prognostic significance of dysrhythmias and of efficacy control of antiarrhythmic therapy, respectively.

Table 1. Detection of ventricular extrasystoles (*VES*) with 24-h ambulatory ECG monitoring in comparison to exercise stress testing in 93 chronic patients with documented coronary artery disease (same group as shown in Fig. 2)

		Ambulatory ECG monitoring						
	VES	Ø		Uniform		Complex		Σ
Exercise stress testing	Ø	7	8%	14	15%	40	43%	61 66%
	Uniform	0		2	2%	16	17%	18 19%
	Complex	1	1%	3	3%	10	11%	14 15%
	Σ	8	9%	19	20%	66	71%	93 100%

Visual Versus Computer-Aided Analysis of Tapes

In view of the high diagnostic sensitivity of ambulatory ECG monitoring, the question arises: What prevented common use of this method after its introduction by Holter 20 years ago [13]? The time spent analyzing 10- to 24-h tapes might have been one reason. The other problem was the significant loss of information caused by visual high-speed tape analysis, the replay unit running at sixty times real time (60:1). This is elucidated by the poor correlation (r = 0.68) between high-speed (60:1) and real-time analysis (1:1) of ventricular extrasystoles in one of our studies, which means that more than 50% (52%) of ectopics are missed by visual high-speed analysis [3, 4, 6]. For these reasons the most significant improvement in Holter technology was the introduction of arrhythmia computers in recent years [26, 27].

In another study we compared incidence and maximal grade of ventricular dysrhythmias in two groups of coronary patients (Figs. 3 and 4). Results of the first group, consisting of 67 coronary patients, were published in 1977 [5]. Until that time we analyzed our long-term ECG tapes visually. In the second group with 170 chronic coronary patients, rhythm analysis was done with the aid of a hybrid computer (Pathfinder II & CBS module) as mentioned above.

Both groups showed a comparable sex distribution, the second group having a slightly higher mean age. Furthermore, the extent of coronary artery disease with regard to the number of significantly obstructed vessels involved did not differ between both groups (stenosis > 75%, single-, double- or triple-vessel disease) (Table 2). Finally, a comparable incidence of normokinetic, hypokinetic, and akinetic left ventricles, respectively, was found in both groups (Table 2). Thus, differences in ectopic activity between these groups should mainly be due to the mode of tape analysis.

In fact, we detected more ectopics by support of the computer (Fig. 3), only 6% (11/170) being free of ectopic activity in the second group, in contrast to 18% (12/67) in the first group. The overall difference between both groups — taking all figures into account by means of multifield-χ^2-analysis — was close to the level of significance ($0.10 > P > 0.05$)

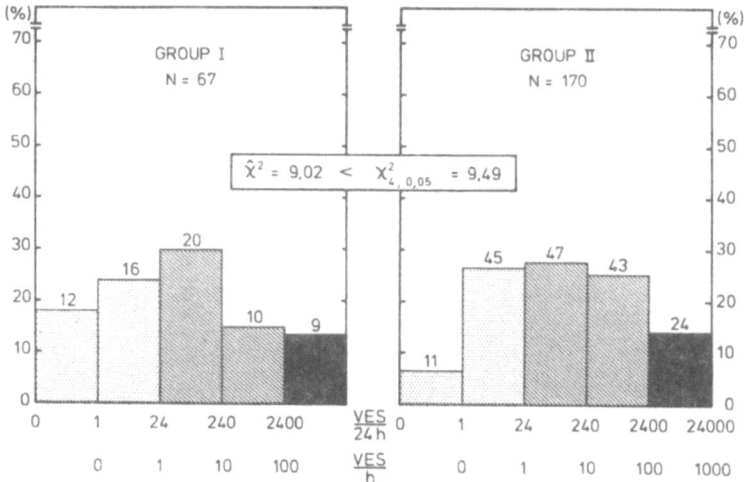

Fig. 3. Comparison of the frequency of ventricular extrasystoles (VES) in two groups of chronic coronary patients, in whom tape analysis of ambulatory ECG monitoring was done visually (Group I; N = 67) and with the aid of an arrhythmia computer, respectively (Group II; N = 170). $\hat{\chi}^2$ = 9.02 = test statistics including all numbers of patients. χ^2_4; 0.05 = 9.49 = tabulated chi-square referring to a degree of freedom of 4 and a level of significance of 5%

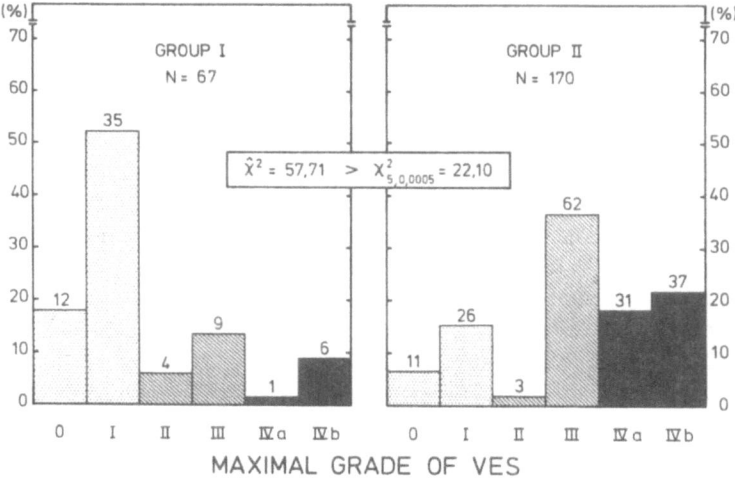

Fig. 4. Comparison of the maximal grade of ventricular extrasystoles (VES) according to Lown's definition [19] in two groups of chronic coronary patients, in whom tape analysis was done visually (Group I; N = 67) and with the aid of an arrhythmia computer, respectively (Group II; N = 170). $\hat{\chi}^2$ = 57.71 = test statistics including all numbers of patients. χ^2_5; 0.0005 = 22.10 = tabulated chi-square referring to a degree of freedom of 5 and a level of significance of 0.05%

Table 2. Comparison of age and sex distribution as well as extent of coronary artery disease (no. of diseased vessels involved; stenosis > 75%) and left ventricular wall motion in two groups of patients, in whom tape analysis of ambulatory ECG monitoring was done visually (Group I; N = 67) and with the aid of an arrhythmia computer, respectively (Group II; N = 170)

24-h ECG monitoring	Group 1 Visual analysis	Group 2 Computer-aided analysis	Statistics
No. of patients	67	170	Σ 237
Male/female	64/3	161/9	ns
Mean age (± SD)	48.7 ± 6.7	51.4 ± 7.5	p < 0.05
Years (range)	36−65	32−69	
MO/1/2/3	10/20/15/22	15/72/48/35	ns
NOR/HYP/AKI	8/12/47	23/29/118	ns

Statistics: Multifield-χ^2-analysis was used to compare incidences of both groups; unpaired t-test was used to compare mean age of both groups; *ns*, not significant; *SD*, standard deviation; *MO*, mild obstructions (stenosis < 75%); 1/2/3 = one, two, or three vessel disease (stenosis > 75%); *NOR*, normokinesis; *HYP*, hypokinesis; *AKI*, akinesis of left ventricle

(Fig. 3). Real time visual analysis (1:1) of the hour of peak incidence of ectopics in the first group obviously prevented significant underestimation of VES frequency.

Even more striking is the difference between both groups with regard to complex forms of ventricular extrasystoles using Lown's maximal grading (Fig. 4). A three- to fourfold higher incidence of class III and class IV arrhythmias were detected in the group in which a computer aided scanning system for tape analysis was used ($P < 0.0005$). In conclusion, computer-aided analysis of magnetic tapes significantly increases diagnostic sensitivity of ambulatory ECG monitoring, since visual analysis depends greatly on the concentration of the examining person and varies accordingly.

Using such a computer-aided scanning system the clinician is interested in two characteristics of the computer which are important in order to obtain reliable results: Sensitivity and specificity. The hybrid computer introduced by Neilson 10 years ago [26], which is part of the Pathfinder used in our studies, was tested by five different groups comparing results of automatic analysis with reading continuous recordings during the same period of time [16, 17, 20, 22, 27]. The results of these independent studies are summarized in Table 3, indicating sensitivity and specificity of the computer as they exceed 90% in all instances. Thus, given a good quality ECG signal, the results obtained with this computer are reliable.

However, artifact detection and suppression still remain inadequate in most computer systems. Figure 5 shows a typical example of this problem. The event module of the computer indicated "pause" in this case. The small and sharp spike following the third QRS complex indicates intermittent loose connection, which is confirmed by the simultaneous dual channel recording; the signal transmission in the upper tracing is restored within milliseconds, an interruption becoming evident only when the signal in the lower tacing happened to be restored already. Thus, we rejected this "pause" as a false positive event.

Since artifacts are common findings in ambulatory ECG monitoring and cannot be completely avoided by careful preparation of the patient and recorder, validation of automatically obtained results by reading ECG tracings is mandatory in order not to draw erroneous

Table 3. Sensitivity and specificity of automatically detected abnormally shaped QRS complexes by means of Neilson's arrhythmia computer (Pathfinder, Reynolds Medical, Hertford, England) [26, 27]

No. of tapes	Tape speed	Sensitivity (%)	Specificity (%)	Author	
29	60:1	97		Neilson, JMM	(1974)
10	1:1	90,9	98,5	Kühn, P	(1976)
25	60:1	0,89[a]		McLeod, A	(1977)
5	60:1	> 97	> 99	Møller, M	(1978)
37	60:1	95,3	97,2	Leitner, ERv	(1981)

[a] Correlation coefficient (automatic analysis in relation to visual real time analysis)

conclusions. In our laboratory complex dysrhythmias such as multiform ectopics and bigeminal rhythm, all consecutive forms of ventricular extrasystoles, and also all R-R intervals exceeding 2 s are routinely validated. As the example in Fig. 5 demonstrates, the specificity of validation increases with dual channel recordings of the ECG.

At Which Stage of Coronary Heart Disease is Ambulatory ECG Recording Helpful?

No follow-up data are available regarding the incidence of ventricular dysrhythmias recorded before and after acute transmural myocardial infarction. But there are several studies dealing with the relationship between angiographic findings and ectopic activity in chronic coronary patients [3, 5, 8, 9, 18, 30, 31]. The authors agree that there is a close relationship between the occurrence of left ventricular akinetic wall motion and frequent ventricular extrasystoles and their complex forms, respectively.

Likewise, in the 170 patients with documented coronary heart disease (group II - Table 2, Figs. 2 and 3) ventricular ectopics showed no relationship to the number of diseased vessels (stenosis > 75%) but to left ventricular impairment. The 118 patients with poststenotic left ventricular akinesis revealed significantly more ectopics within 24 h than 29 patients with regional hypokinesis or 23 patients with still normal wall motility ($P < 0.01$; Fig. 6). With regard to the maximal grading of ventricular extrasystoles following Lown's definition, a similar correlation was found between the reduction of left ventricular wall motion and increasing incidence of complex ventricular dysrhythmias ($P < 0.005$; Fig. 7). The incidence of dysrhythmias was independent of the localization of akinetic areas, which involved the anterior wall 72 times and the inferior wall 46 times. This suggests that the mere presence of ischemia-damaged myocardium constitutes the condition for enhanced triggered automaticity and reentry mechanism, respectively, thereby increasing the probability of ectopic activity.

These findings imply that predominantly patients after transmural myocardial infarction represent a target group for detailed rhythm analysis. Thus, the posthospital phase of acute myocardial infarction, in which many patients undergo cardiac rehabilitation, is a most rewarding period for ambulatory ECG monitoring in order to recognize ectopic activity in patients being at increased risk for sudden cardiac death. According to the high mortality rate, especially in the early posthospital phase of transmural myocardial infarction [24, 25],

♂ V.H. 57 years old   LZ-EKG 102/80

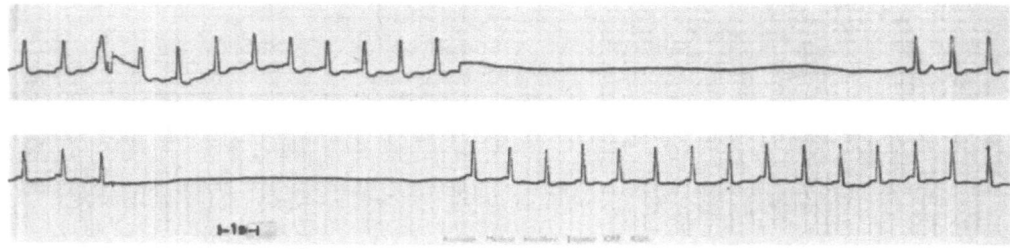

Fig. 5. Simultaneous dual channel ECG recording from a 57-year-old male patient suffering from coronary heart disease. The event module of the arrhythmia computer indicated "pause" during this episode. For further details see text

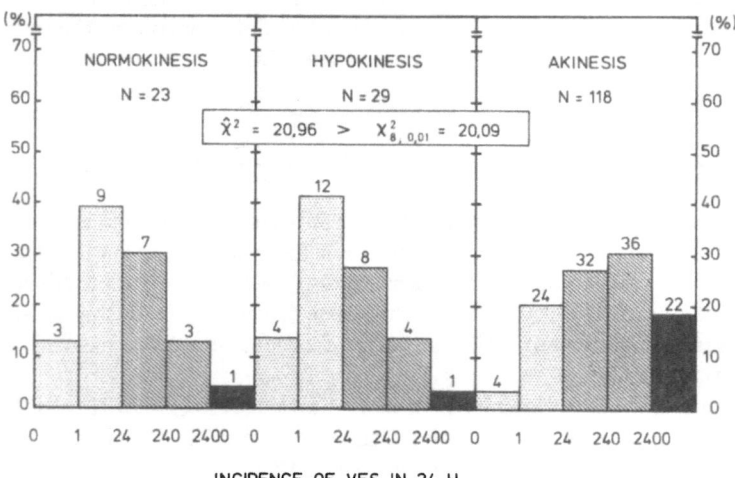

INCIDENCE OF VES IN 24 H

Fig. 6. Incidence of ventricular extrasystoles (VES) within 24-h monitoring periods in relation to left ventricular wall motion in 170 chronic coronary patients (identical with Group II in Table 2, Figs. 3 and 4). $\hat{\chi}^2 = 20.96$ = test statistics including all numbers of patients. χ^2_8; 0.01 = 20.09 = tabulated chi-square referring to a degree of freedom of 8 and a level of significance of 1%

only early cardiac rehabilitation, as well as early careful rhythm control, may contribute to a reduction in sudden coronary deaths. Furthermore, ambulatory ECG monitoring is not only a helpful tool for diagnostic reasons at this stage of coronary heart disease, but is also mandatory in patients receiving antiarrhythmic therapy since the effect of a given drug cannot be predicted from its electrophysiologic properties [4].

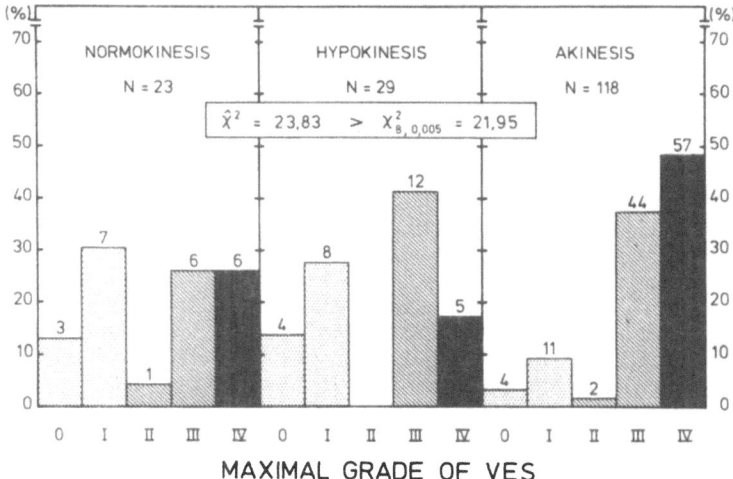

Fig. 7. Maximal grade of ventricular extrasystoles according to Lown's definition [19] in relation to left ventricular wall motion in 170 chronic coronary patients (identical with Group II in Table 2, Figs. 3 and 4). $\hat{\chi}^2 = 23.83$ = test statistics including all numbers of patients. χ^2_8; 0.005 = 21.95 = tabulated chi-square referring to a degree of freedom of 8 and a level of significance of 0.5%

Summary

Ambulatory ECG monitoring is a very sensitive method for assessing spontaneous incidence of dysrhythmias. With the introduction of arrhythmia computers this diagnostic sensitivity was improved further, but automatic artifact detection and suppression remains a problem to be solved. For this reason, validation of dysrhythmias with prognostic implications is mandatory in order to separate true positive from false positive events.

Ambulatory ECG monitoring has proved to be a helpful tool, especially in patients with coronary heart disease. The significant relationship between akinetic wall motion and increased ectopic activity indicates that patients after acute myocardial infarction represent a target group for detailed rhythm analysis, a fact which can be used to characterize patients with increased risk of sudden cardiac death. Despite the lack of evidence that antiarrhythmic therapy improves prognosis in postinfarction patients with serious dysrhythmias, it is essential to check the effect of medication with rhythm analysis in view of the unpredictable effectiveness of the drugs as well as in view of the unpredictable moment of sudden cardiac death.

References

1 Andresen D, Tietze U, von Leitner ER, Lehmann HU, Thormann I, Wessel HJ, Schröder R (1980) Spontanvariabilität tachykarder Rhythmusstörungen. Z Kardiol 69:214
2 Bertel O, Braun S, Schmid P, Burkart F (1979) Hohe Spontanvariabilität ventrikulärer Rhythmusstörungen limitiert Aussagekraft von Langzeit-EKG-Untersuchungen. Schweiz Med Wochenschr 109:1670−1672
3 Bethge K-P, Lichtlen PR (1979) Ventricular arrhythmias in relation to the extent of coronary lesions and left ventricular function. In: MacFarlane PW (ed) Progress in electrocardiology. Pitman, London, p 126
4 Bethge K-P, Lichtlen PR (1981) Die Beurteilung der antiarrhythmischen Therapie durch Langzeit-Elektrokardiographie. In: Lüderitz B (ed) Ventrikuläre Herzrhythmusstörungen. Springer, Berlin Heidelberg New York, p 170
5 Bethge K-P, Bethge H-C, Graf A, van den Berg E, Lichtlen P (1977) Kammer-Arrhythmien bei chronisch koronarer Herzkrankheit. Analyse anhand des Langzeit-Elektrokardiogrammes und der selektiven Koronarangiographie bzw. linksventrikulären Angiographie. Z Kardiol 66:1−9
6 Bethge K-P, Godt U, Lichtlen PR (1977) Zur Frage der computerunabhängigen quantitativen Auswertung von ambulanten Langzeit-EKG. Biomed Techn (Suppl) 22:199−200
7 Bühlmann A (1975) Probleme und Erfahrungen mit der Ergometrie in der klinischen Praxis. In: Mellerowicz H, Jokl E, Hansen G (eds) Ergebnisse der Ergometrie. Perimed, Erlangen, p 193
8 Califf RM, Burks JM, Behar VS, Margolis JR, Wagner GS (1978) Relationships among ventricular arrhythmias, coronary artery disease, and angiographic and electrocardiographic indicators of myocardial fibrosis. Circulation 57:725−732
9 Calvert A, Lown B, Gorlin R (1977) Ventricular premature beats and anatomically defined coronary heart disease. Am J Cardiol 39:627−634
10 Crawford M, O'Rourke RA, Ramakrishna N, Henning H, Ross J (1974) Comparative effectiveness of exercise testing and continuous monitoring for detecting arrhythmias in patients with previous myocardial infarction. Circulation 50:301−305
11 van Durme JP, Pannier R (1978) Prevalence and prognostic significance of ventricular dysrhythmias during the first year after myocardial infarction. In: Mäurer W, Schömig A, Dietz R, Lichten PR (eds) Beta-Blockade 1977, Thieme, Stuttgart, p 286
12 Fitzgerald JW, de Busk RF (1975) Early post-infarction ambulatory monitoring and exercise testing in detection of arrhythmias. Am J Cardiol 35:136
13 Holter NJ (1961) New method for heart studies. Science 134:1214−1220
14 Kennedy HL, Chandra V, Sayther KL, Caralis DG (1978) Effectiveness of increasing hours of continuous ambulatory electrocardiography in detecting maximal ventricular ectopy. Am J Cardiol 42:925−930
15 Kosowsky BD, Lown B, Whiting R, Guiney T (1971) Occurrence of ventricular arrhythmias with exercise as compared to monitoring. Circulation 44:826−832
16 Kühn P, Kroiss A, Joskowicz G (1976) Arrhythmieanalyse − Arrhythmieüberwachung. (Vergleichsuntersuchungen von 4 Kleincomputern zur automatischen EKG-Überwachung). Z Kardiol 65:166−175
17 Leitner ER von, Tietze U, Andresen D, Schröder R (1981) Rechnerkompatibles Langzeit-EKG-Analysegerät zur quantitativen Erfassung einfacher und komplexer Rhythmusstörungen; Systembeschreibung und Untersuchung der Analysegenauigkeit. Z Kardiol 70:22−27
18 Lichtlen PR, Bethge K-P, Platiel P (1980) Inzidenz des plötzlichen Herztodes bei Koronarpatienten in Abhängigkeit von Anatomie und Rhythmusprofil. Z Kardiol 69:639−648
19 Lown B, Wolf M (1971) Approaches to sudden death from coronary heart disease. Circulation 44:130−142
20 McLeod A, Kitson D, McComish M, Jewitt D (1977) Role of ambulatory electrocardiographic monitoring; accuracy of quantitative analysis system. Br Heart J 39:347

21 Michelson EL, Morganroth J (1980) Spontaneous variability of complex ventricular arrhythmias detected by long-term electrocardiographic recording. Circulation 61: 690–695

22 Møller M (1978) Reliability of quantitative analysis of ambulatory ECG tape recordings. Trans Eur Soc Cardiol 1:30

23 Morganroth J, Michelson EL, Horowitz LN, Josephson ME, Pearlman AS, Dunkman WB (1978) Limitations of routine long-term electrocardiographic monitoring to assess ventricular ectopic frequency. Circulation 58:408–414

24 Moss AJ, Decamilla J, Mietlowski W, Greene WA, Goldstein S, Locksley R (1975) Prognostic grading and significance of ventricular premature beats after recovery from myocardial infarction. Circulation (Suppl III) 52:204–210

25 Moss AJ, Decamilla JJ, Davis HP, Bayer L (1977) Clinical significance of ventricular ectopic beats in the early posthospital phase of myocardial infarction. Am J Cardiol 39:635–640

26 Neilson JMM (1971) A special purpose hybrid computer for analysis of ECG arrhythmias. IEE Conf Publ, London 79:151

27 Neilson JMM (1974) High speed analysis of ventricular arrhythmias from 24 hour recordings. Comput Cardiol 74 CH 0379–7C:55–61

28 Ruberman W, Weinblatt E, Frank CW, Goldberg JD, Shapiro S, Feldman CL (1975) Ventricular premature beats and mortality of men with coronary heart disease. Circulation (Suppl III) 52:199–201

29 Ryan M, Lown B, Horn H (1975) Comparison of ventricular ectopic activity during 24 hour monitoring and exercise testing in patients with coronary heart disease. N Engl J Med 292:224–229

30 Samek L, Kirste D, Roskamm H, Stürzenhofecker P, Prokoph J (1977) Herzrhythmusstörungen nach Herzinfarkt. Herz Kreislauf 9:641–649

31 Simon H, Gross-Fengels W, Schilling G, Schaede A (1980) Ventrikuläre Rhythmusstörungen im ambulanten Langzeit-EKG in Abhängigkeit vom Befund im Belastungs-EKG. Herz Kreislauf 12:103–110

32 Tietze U, Leitner ER von, Andresen D, Schröder R (1979) Ein Langzeit-EKG-Analysesystem zur quantitativen Auswertung von Herzrhythmusstörungen. Biomed Tech 24: 275–280

33 Vorpahl U, Blümchen G (1978) Supraventrikuläre und ventrikuläre Extrasystolen bei Patienten in der späten Postinfarktphase. Z Kardiol 67:612–620

34 Winkle RA (1978) Antiarrhythmic drug effect mimicked by spontaneous variability of ventricular ectopy. Circulation 57:1116–1121

ECG Telemetry

K. Bachmann

Today four methods are available for laboratory remote recording of the ECG. Due to the difficulties involved in bringing patients to the laboratory, as early as 1906 Einthoven developed a phone transmission apparatus, the Telecardiogramme, in order to record ECG with a string galvanometer at a distance form the hospital [7]. Radiotransmission of the ECG was the next step introduced by Holter before he started to "uninvent" the radio link by recording with the Elektrocardiocorder on tape [8—10]. Holter monitoring is now commonly in use and has become the number one method in use for ambulatory monitoring. Furthermore solid state recording facilitates intermittent storage-telemetry of ECG-derived information such as heart rate and arrhythmia (Fig. 1).

ECG telemetry, which was primarily focused on measuring R-R intervals, was first applied to record heart rate and detect arrhythmias. This was achieved by a lower standard of technology in comparison with currently available methods, which make possible computer-assisted analysis not only of the QRS complex but also of the ST segment. Every method of ambulatory or long distance recording of the ECG has its advantages and disadvantages, making it superior in different fields of application or, in the view of Holter, "Radiotelemetry is needed for some situations and storage-telemetry for others" [11].

Radiotransmission of the ECG never had the technical problem of direct coupling of the ECG signal which was encountered during portable tape recording. The frequency modulation of the ECG provided the opportunity, from the very beginning, for detection not only of myocardial electrical instability but also of myocardial ischemia from ST segment changes. However, nowadays the second generation of tape recording of the frequency modulated signal, with a bandwidth of 0.05—100 Hz (AHA specification) has overcome these differences between radiotransmission and Holter monitoring. Recent advances in technology, introducing a conceptually new approach, have resulted in the development of preprocessing and event recorders which improve analysis of arrhythmias and myocardial ischemia as far as data reduction, recognition accuracy, and documentation are concerned [14, 16, 21, 22].

Moreover, transmission of the ECG by radio offers the advantage of monitoring the patient on a scope simultaneously. This makes ECG telemetry superior to other methods of ambulatory ECG monitoring in patients at risk during rehabilitation of everyday hemodynamic stress and the cardiovascular response to it. Thus ECG telemetry is especially appropriate in monitoring patients who are at risk during exposure to both physical and emotional stress. Simultaneous monitoring under these conditions is provided by radiotransmission only.

A third advantage is the greater technical versatility of ECG telemetry by radiotransmission. Multichannel systems with programmable preamplifiers are capable of transmitting not only the ECG but also other cardiovascular parameters, for example, pressure from the arterial system and the pulmonary artery simultaneously [2—4, 26]. This provides the facility of measuring everyday hemodynamic stress in terms of preload, afterload, left ventricular performance, and the doubleproduct [19], which is the major indicator of myocardial oxygen demand.

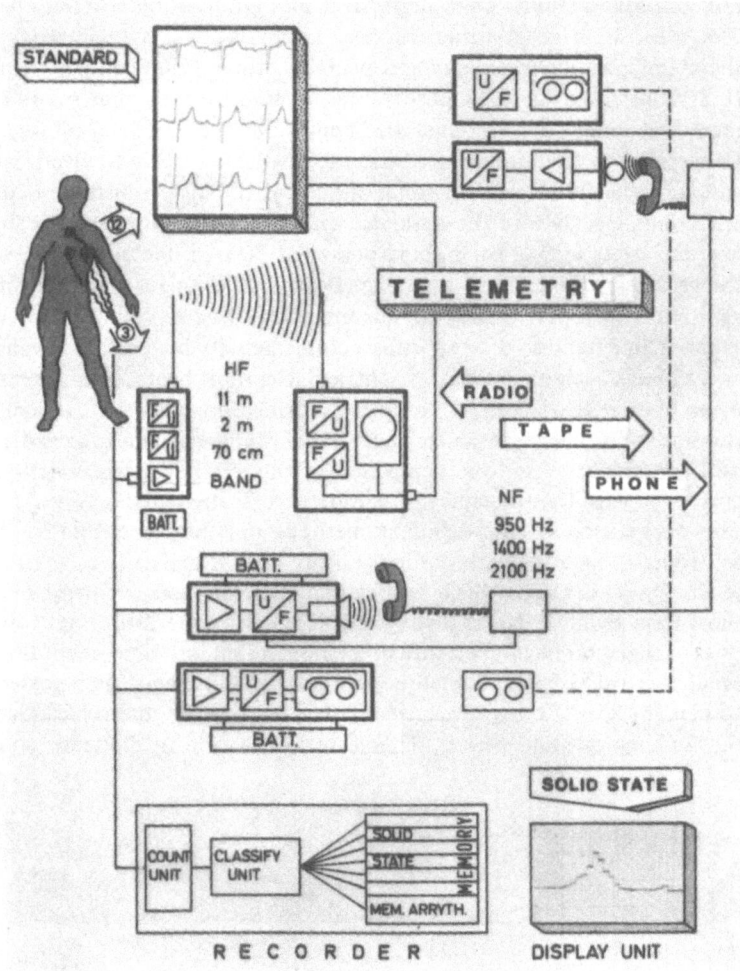

Fig. 1. Block diagram of laboratory remote ECG recording by radio, phone, tape, and solid state

To define the field of application of ECG telemetry in coronary heart disease one has to bear in mind that much of the ground covered by radiotelemetry formerly has now been taken over by tape recording. There are still special circumstances where radiotransmission using frequency modulation or pulse code modulation is appropriate. The problem lies in finding which form of the ECG recording is most appropriate to: first, myocardial ischemia and electrical instability: second, the estimation of everyday hemodynamic stress and cardiovascular response to it; and third, providing guidance in primary and secondary prevention during physical activity and training.

We approached these questions insofar as coronary insufficiency and arrhythmias are concerned by comparing standard exercise testing with the 24-h tape recording and radiotransmission. These studies were performed in a group of 69 coronary patients with a more than 75% stenosis in at least one coronary artery [4, 17]. Exercise stress testing on a bicycle in the sitting position was the most sensitive method of indicating ischemic ST segment changes. It demonstrated an 87% positive result compared to that of 49% during radiotelemetry recording under "open-air-exercise" conditions and 35% by 24-h tape recording (Fig. 2).

Conversely, in the more prognostic tool of the detection of electrical instability of the myocardium, the 24-h tape recording method is the most sensitive. It demonstrates ventricular arrhythmias in 97% of the patients, while the 4-h radiotelemetry shows only 83%. Further exercise stress testing for a short period of 30 min, including a 10-minute recovery period, shows a mere 51%. Thus we conclude that the longer the time of observation the more ventricular ectopic activity is documented. Tape recording showed itself to be not only superior in detection of ventricular ectopic activity but also of advanced forms of ventricular arrhythmias such as multifocal ventricular ectopic beats, couplets, salvos and R-on-T phenomena (Lown III–V [15]). There is a correlation between the incidence of ventricular arrhythmias and left ventricular angiographic findings. The type and extent of left ventricular wall abnormalities and the depression of the left ventricular ejection fraction are positively correlated with the frequency of ectopic ventricular activity (Fig. 3).

The comparison of the different methods presently available for laboratory-remote ECG recording in patients with coronary heart disease makes it clear that the sensitivity of ECG telemetry in detecting both myocardial ischemia and electrical instability lies in between short-term exercise stress testing and long-term tape recording. Our group of coronary patients, angiographically classified, demonstrated on tape recording tests not such a high predictive value in the detection of myocardial ischemia as reported by other documented studies [6, 23–25]. However, we think this could be due to differences in workload during the 24-h monitoring period. Therefore in the field of diagnosis and prognosis of coronary

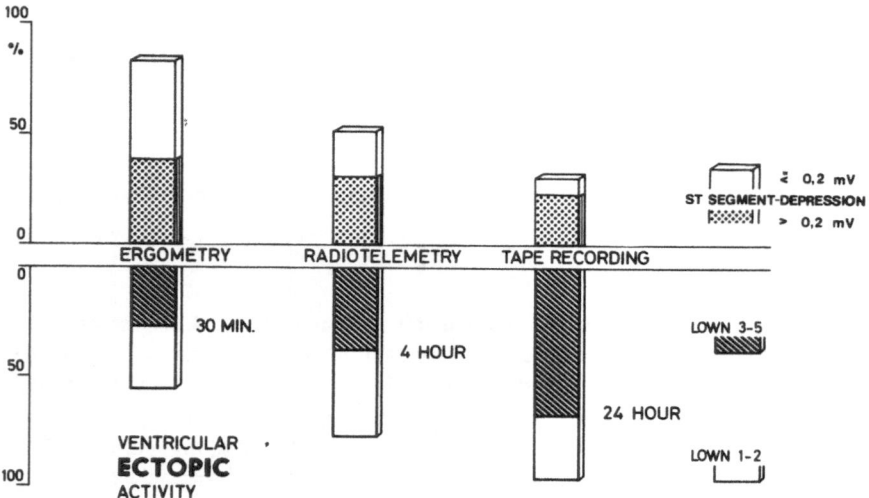

Fig. 2. Results of standard exercise testing radioelemetry and 24-h tape recording in detecting myocardial ischemia and electrical instability in 96 patients with angiographically documented coronary heart disease

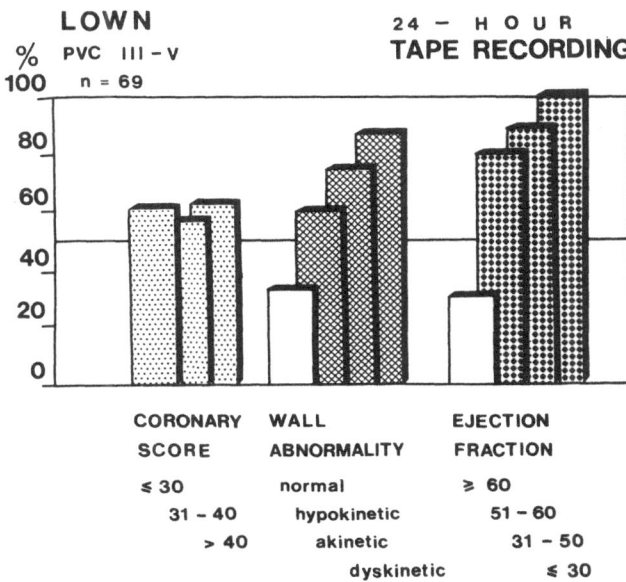

Fig. 3. Influence of myocardial ischemia (coronary score), scar tissue (wall abnormalities), and left ventricular pump function (ejection fraction) on the incidence of ventricular ectopic activity in patients with coronary heart disease

heart disease, ECG telemetry is of little help and gives us no additional information over and above the exercise stress testing and Holter monitoring.

The most important use of ECG telemetry lies in guarding the patient at risk during everyday activities. This application mainly deals with rehabilitation after myocardial infarction and primary and secondary prevention of coronary heart disease [13, 20, 24]. Furthermore, information on everyday hemodynamic stress and cardiovascular response to it is provided by ambulatory monitoring only [5, 12, 18]. In this field radiotransmission of cardiovascular parameters may be of real help and preferable to tape recording and transmission by phone. This is because it makes possible the simultaneous monitoring of the patient on a scope, a prerequisite in combined studies with simultaneous blood pressure measurements in the systemic and pulmonary circulation [2–4, 26]. Therefore ECG telemetry has its major application in the ambulatory monitoring of both the patient at risk and under hemodynamic stress when information on myocardial ischemia or electrical instability is needed immediately. Such situations may arise either during rehabilitation or during exposure to extreme demands such as high altitude hypoxemia, physical training by swimming, and isometric exercise.

Analyzing hemodynamic stress by ECG telemetry exclusively has been overemphazied in the past insofar as the heart rate profile as a workload indicator is concerned. Simultaneous registration of heart rate and arterial blood pressure has demonstrated remarkably differences in heart rate profile during dynamic, isometric, and combined physical stress. Heart rate as a workload indicator is reliable in dynamic physical activity only but may mislead completely in isometric exercise or in situations such as swimming or gymnastics prescribed

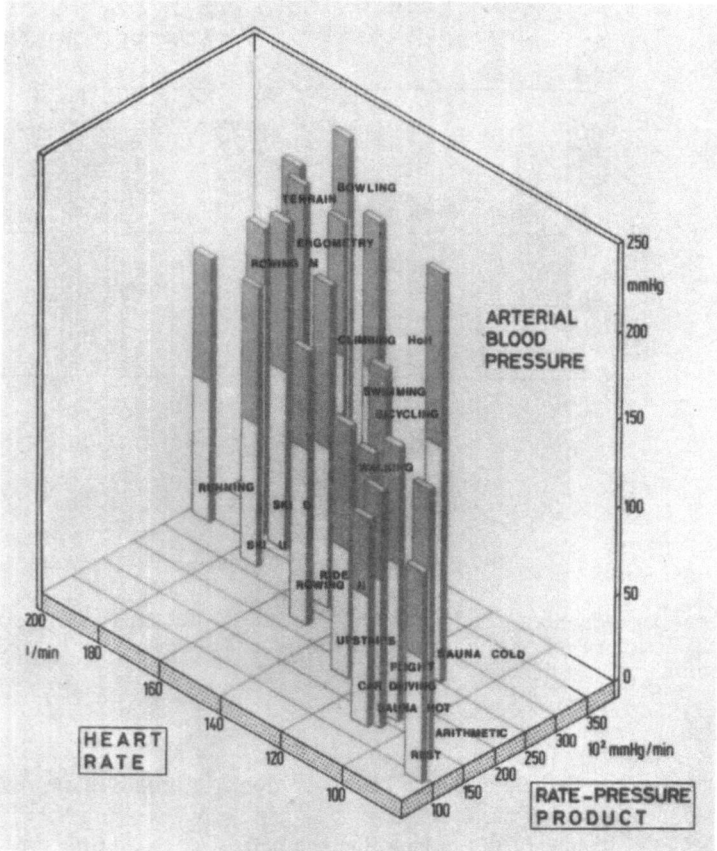

Fig. 4. Hemodynamic stress of everyday situation and sport activities in terms of arterial pressure and heart rate as indicated by radiotelemetry of ECG and continuous intra-arterial blood pressure measurements. Heart rate per se indicates afterload (arterial pressure) and myocardial oxygen demand (pressure rate product) in dynamic exercise only and may mislead completely in evaluating isometric workload

for rehabilitation purposes. Thus simultaneous telemetry of the ECG and arterial pressure has given new information on everyday hemodynamic stress which may serve as a guideline· for maximal physical training at a minimal risk. This in turn can be used as a preventive measure in healthy subjects at risk and in the rehabilitation of the cardiac patient (Fig. 4).

Summary. Today ECG telemetry is chiefly concerned with basic clinical research, leaving the field of diagnosis and prognosis to standard exercise testing or 24-h Holter monitoring. The technology of radiotransmission makes ECG telemetry superior in situations which require simultaneous monitoring of the subject or combined recording of the ECG with other cardiovascular parameters such as pulmonary artery and systemic blood pressure. Thus ECG telemetry may be best applied either in the rehabilitation of patients at risk or in the monitoring of subjects exposed to extreme hemodynamic stress.

References

1 Allen RD, Geltes LS, Phalan C, Avington D (1976) Painless ST-segment depression in patients with angina pectoris. Chest 69:467
2 Bachmann K, Thebis J (1967) Die drahtlose Übertragung kontinuierlicher, direkter Blutdruckmessungen. Z Kreislaufforsch 56:188
3 Bachmann K, Thebis J (1968) Die telefonische Übermittlung direkter kontinuierlicher Blutdruckmessungen. Z Kreislaufforsch 57:290
4 Bachmann K (1981) The value of telemetry. In: Loogen F, Seipel L (eds) Detection of ischemic myocardium with exercise. Springer, Berlin Heidelberg New York (in press)
5 Blatter K, Imhof P (1969) Die Rolle der adrenergen Beta-Rezeptoren bei emtionellen Tachykardie; radiotelemetrische Untersuchungen an Skispringern. Schweiz Sportmed 17:131
6 Crawford MH, Mendoza CA, O'Rourke RA, White DH, Boucher CA, Gorwith J (1978) Limitations of continuous electrocardiogram monitoring for detection of coronary artery disease. Ann Int Med 89:1
7 Einthoven W (1906) The telecardiogramme. Arch Internal Physiol 4:132
8 Holter NJ (1957) Radioelectrocardiography: A new technique for cardiovascular studies. Ann NY Acad Scie 913
9 Holter NJ (1972) Storage telemetry and sudden death. In: Kimmich HP, Voss A (eds) Biotelemetry. Meander, Leiden
10 Holter NJ (1980) Real-time analysis of Holter ECG data represents a major technological advance. Holter Res Found Bull Febr
11 Holter NJ, Gengerelli JA (1949) Remote recording of physiological data by radio. Rocky Mt Med J 46:747
12 Imhof P, Blatter K, Imhof U, Howald H, Turri M (1971) Radiotelemetrische Herzfrequenzmessungen an Skilangläufern. Schweiz Z Sportmed 19:27
13 Kalusche D, Samek L, Roskamm H (1981) ECG telemetry in the ambulatory monitoring of the cardiac patient during rehabilitation. Biotelemetry and patient monitoring (in press)
14 Kimmich HP (1981) Portable solid-state recorder for long-term assessment of physiological parameters in form of a histogram. Biotelemetry and patient monitoring (in press)
15 Lown B, Wolf M (1971) Approaches to sudden death from coronary heart disease. Circulation 44:130
16 Morris JRW, Simpson AF (1980) Ambulatory tape recording. In: Littler WA (ed) Clinical ambulatory monitoring. Chapman and Hall, London, pp 1–26
17 Raab G, Bachmann K, Zerzawy R, Dalianis N (1981) Ambulatory monitoring of ventricular arrhythmias and ischemia in coronary patients. Comparison of radiotelemetry and type recordings. In: Matsumoto G, Kimmich HP (eds) Biotelemetry V. Matsumoto and Kimmich, Sapporo-Njimegen
18 Reid DH, Doerr JE (1970) Physiological studies of military parachutists via FM/FM telemetry: the data aquisition system and heart rate response. Aerospace Medicine 41:1292
19 Robinson BF (1967) Relation of heart rate and systolic blood pressure to the onset of pain in angina pectoris. Circulation 35:1073
20 Samek L, Roskamm H (1977) EKG-Telemetrie in der Rehabilitation von Infarktkranken. Biomed Technik 22:183
21 Saris WHM, Snel P, Baecke J, van Waesberghe F, Binkhorst RA (1977) A portable miniature solid-state heart rate recorder for monitoring daily physical activity. Biotelemetry 4:131
22 Simons ML, Boehmer T, Roelandt J (1981) The value of Holter monitoring for detection of ischemic heart disease. In: Loogen F, Seipel L (eds) Detection of ischemic myocardium. Springer, Berlin Heidelberg New York (in press)
23 Stern S, Tzivoni D (1974) Early detection of silent ischemic heart disease by 24-hour electrocardiographic monitoring in active subjects. Br Heart J 36:481–486

24   Stern S, Tzivoni D, Stern Z (1975) Diagnostic accuracy of ambulatory ECG-monitoring in ischemic heart disease. Circulation 52:1045
25   Wolf E, Tzivoni D, Stern S (1974) Comparison of exercise test and 24-hour ambulatory electrocardiographic monitoring in detection of ST-T changes. Br Heart J 36:90
26   Zerzawy R, Bachmann K (1974) A programmable four channel system for long-time radiotelemetry of biomedical parameters. In: Kimmich HP, Voss JA (eds) Biotelemetry, Meander, Leiden, p 49

Subject Index

Of Further Interest:

Comprehensive Manuals of Surgical Specialties

Editor: R. H. Egdahl

B. J. Harlan, A. Starr, F. M. Harwin

Manual of Cardiac Surgery

Volume 1
1980. 193 figures (183 full in color), 8 tables. XV, 204 pages
ISBN 3-540-90393-3

B. J. Harlan, A. Starr, F. M. Harwin

Manual of Cardiac Surgery

Volume 2
1981. 130 figures in full color. XV, 143 pages
ISBN 3-540-90563-4

Frontiers in Hypertension Research

Editors: J. H. Laragh, F. R. Bühler, D. W. Seldin
1981. 246 figures. XXXIX, 628 pages
ISBN 3-540-90557-X
Distribution rights for Japan: Igaku Shoin, Tokyo

The Heart in Hypertension

Editor: B. E. Strauer
1981. 187 figures, 55 tables. XVI, 464 pages
(International Boehringer Mannheim Symposia)
ISBN 3-540-10496-8

Hypertension: Mechanisms and Management

Editors: T. Philipp, A. Distler
1980. 72 figures, 17 tables. XVII, 279 pages (23 pages in German)
(International Boehringer Mannheim Symposia)
ISBN 3-540-10171-3

Hypertrophic Cardiomyopathy

The Therapeutic Role of Calcium Antagonists
Editors: M. Kaltenbach, S. E. Epstein
1981. 172 figures, approx. 46 tables. Approx. 368 pages
ISBN 3-540-11065-8

Myocardial Infarction at Young Age

International Symposium Held in Bad Krozingen, January 30th
and 31th, 1981
Editor: H. Roskamm
198 . 83 figures. Approx. 240 pages
ISBN 3-540-11090-9

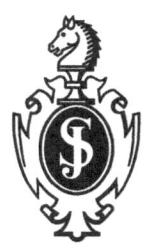

Springer-Verlag
Berlin
Heidelberg
New York

Myocardial Infarction and Psychosocial Risks

Editors: J. Siegrist, M. J. Halhuber
With contributions by numerous experts

1981. 23 figures, 33 tables. X, 152 pages
ISBN 3-540-10386-4

This volume contains contributions presented at the Fourth International Workshop on Psychosocial Stress and Coronary Heart Disease (CHD) held in Höhenried in July, 1979. Special emphasis is placed on the results of sociological and epidemiological studies linking work stress, chronic and acute conflict, lack of social support and risk attitudes and behaviors (type A behavior) to the onset of myocardial infarction. Psychosocial and psychophysiological contributions point out the mechanisms by which stress can lead cardiovascular damage. The final chapter provides a critical evaluation of the goals and problems of research in this promising interdisciplinary field.

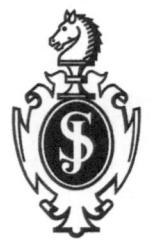

Springer-Verlag
Berlin
Heidelberg
New York